A RATE YOURSELF

Find out how healthy you *really* are

HEALTH IMPROVEMENT PROGRAMS

Relaxation
Cardiovascular fitness
Flexibility
Fun

WEIGHT LOSS

The natural way

HYDROTHERAPY AND HELIOTHERAPY

How to use water and sunlight to strengthen the
nervous system and promote robust health

DIET FOR A SMALL, HAPPY STOMACH

GOOD HOUSEKEEPING

The principles of superior elimination

SKIN CARE AND BEAUTY TIPS

OLD-FASHIONED REMEDIES FOR
MODERN-DAY AILMENTS

THE ART OF A GOOD NIGHT'S SLEEP

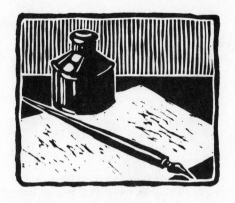

The Art of
Good Living

*Simple Steps
to Regaining Health
and the Joy of Life*

Svevo Brooks

Houghton Mifflin Company   Boston   1990

For information about permission to reproduce selections from
this book, write to Permissions, Houghton Mifflin Company,
2 Park Street, Boston, Massachusetts 02108.

Library of Congress Cataloging-in-Publication Data

Brooks, Svevo.
The art of good living: simple steps to regaining health and the joy
of life / by Svevo Brooks.
p.   cm.
Reprint. Originally published: Capitola, Calif. : Botanica Press,
c 1986.
Includes bibliographical references.
ISBN 0-395-52101-7
1. Health.   2. Natural foods.   3. Youthfulness.   I. Title.
RA776.B777   1989   89-19824
613.2 — dc20   CIP

Printed in the United States of America

D 10 9 8 7 6 5 4 3 2 1

Drawings and woodcuts by Margaret Chodos, except for those on
dedication and pages 40, 42, 102, and 112.

The advice offered in this book is not intended to replace the
care of your family doctor. Its purpose is to teach prevention
and help you, the reader, work better with your doctor and other
health professionals to improve your health.

This book was first published by Botanica Press in 1986 as
Common Sense Diet and Health.

To my grandfather, Louis Brooks,
my inspiration from the past

To my son, Noah Haynes Brooks,
my inspiration for the future

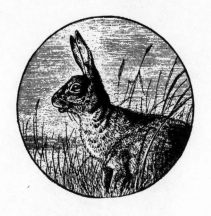

To All Who Appreciate the Wisdom
and Beauty of Nature
And Seek to Emulate Her Healthy Ways

The end of all our exploring will be
to arrive where we started and
know the place for the first time.

— T. S. Eliot

A bit of knowledge gained each day,
In time to wisdom points the way.

— Mother Nature

Contents

Introduction

This is a lovely, important, and truly admirable book. When I first began reading it, I realized at once how special it was and purchased several copies to lend to people who I felt needed its help. But when I returned to those people to see what progress they had made and to take back the book to lend to others, no one wanted to give up his copy! The reason they gave me was always the same: "This book is truly common sense."

This is a book which will last and last because it upholds basic, age-old teachings, in fact biblical ones, which honor the angels of air, light, and water and respect the delicately balanced wholeness of the earth. Living in harmony with nature, which this book teaches so eloquently, is essential for human survival and for the survival of the entire world, including its wonderful fauna and flora.

The seven prescriptions that form the basis for this work are prescriptions for living the truly good life and should be hung in every child's nursery and schoolroom, in offices, public buildings, kitchens — indeed, in all places where humans gather. If these prescriptions were to be followed widely, the world, which at present is threatened and endangered because of an unwise and unnatural lifestyle, would become a happier and safer place for us all.

Juliette de Bairacli Levy
Kythera, Greece

Foreword

Our ancestors, if they were alive today, would surely be amused to see grown men and women running round and round on a track, pedaling stationary bicycles, or doing calisthenics and deep breathing in front of television sets. Their reaction to these special exercises might be very similar to the way some children reacted to me a few years ago when I was jogging on the playground of the local elementary school.

I had jogged in this schoolyard many times before, but always in the evening or on weekends. On this particular day I went jogging in the afternoon and was running alone, quietly absorbed in my own thoughts and footsteps. Suddenly, without warning, the silence of the afternoon was shattered by a crescendo of excited voices. Laughing, shouting, screaming children were everywhere: playing tag, climbing like monkeys on bars and rings, jumping on top of each other's backs, skipping rope, throwing balls, doing somersaults and cartwheels, dashing here and there — all the while hooting and hollering as though they were trying to announce something very important to the rest of the world. As I ran past the swings, one of them asked me what I was doing.

"Exercising," I said, and continued running around the field. The next time I passed, two children jumped off the swings and began running alongside me. "Wanna play?" they asked shyly. I smiled at this childish invitation. "Not now," I said, "gotta finish my run."

We ran together, slowly circling the field, each time joined by a few more laughing and exuberant children. Soon we were five, then seven, and finally a dozen or more. For the first couple of laps the children more or less followed my lead, running beside me, but then they began to zig and zag, then run sideways and occasionally even backward in a kind of follow-the-leader game. At first I ignored these diversions; though amusing, they interfered with the cadence of my running. But the spirit of these children was infectious and I could not long resist the temptation to join in their games. Shyly, but with increasing enthusiasm, I began to follow them and soon found myself skipping, zigzagging, doing somersaults, balancing like a tightrope walker along the top of a cement ledge, hopping on one foot then the other, racing to imaginary candy shops and ice cream stores which rose up like oases in the midst of a vast desert playground.

But then, just as I was beginning to relax and really enjoy this new game, a bell rang. Within seconds the magical field was silent and empty; my laughing, shouting, running friends were gone.

For two or three minutes I stood quietly in the silence, still filled with the laughter and excitement of recess. Then I began slowly jogging around the field again, hearing only the *clomp-clomp* of my own footsteps in the grass. But now the running felt boring and laborious, my legs were heavy and my mind easily distracted. I kept thinking of the children and how much fun I had been having. Everything had been so effortless, so enjoyable. Now, by contrast, each step was a chore. After a few minutes I felt tired and had no incentive to continue; feeling empty and somewhat sad, I walked slowly home.

That afternoon run on the elementary school playground

was like a splash of cold water in the face (more children's games!). I suddenly realized how serious, boring, and ineffectual my own exercise program was compared to the play of children. Why else would they ask me what I was doing? I also began to think about my reasons for exercising. Why should it be necessary to make exercise a special activity with special facilities, clothing, and equipment? Why couldn't I just get my exercise from normal daily living?

The answer was simple: exercise was something I scheduled and planned. It happened on certain days, at certain hours, and in certain prescribed ways. Exercise was a welcome diversion from my normal sedentary activities: it gave me a chance to stretch my muscles, kept my weight down, and got me outdoors, in closer contact with nature.

While the idea of getting exercise as part of daily life was appealing, it seemed unlikely. The only regular exercise provided by my daily routine was for my tongue; eating and talking gave it plenty of exertion. And while I had thoroughly enjoyed those childish moments on the playground, I knew inside that I was not ready for monkey bars, jump ropes, and somersaults — at least not on a regular basis. What I needed was something simpler, more practical and subdued.

Though my own routine — jogging, calisthenics, an occasional swim, some tennis — was enjoyable and to a certain extent relaxing, it was not completely satisfying. It was expensive, took more time than I would have liked, and didn't seem to make me feel that much better. Still, it was the best I could do. Or was it?

I thought about my ancestors, who were probably hunters and gatherers. Surely they didn't exercise. They probably didn't even know the word as we use it today. They didn't join health clubs, eat vitamin pills, or go on special diets. They didn't do situps, lift weights, or run around in circles on a track. They didn't have to. In order to survive, they were constantly moving — crawling under branches, climbing over rocks, lifting, pulling, bending, walking miles and miles every day. In short, they were busy just living their lives.

Moreover, it occurred to me that these "natural" exercises as practiced daily by my ancestors were very similar to our earliest movements. When a baby is born, for example, she kicks her legs in the air and wiggles her toes, hands, arms, and head. In a total way, a baby uses her body from the moment she enters the world — and even long before. As she grows and learns to coordinate and use the different parts of her body, her life becomes a continuous succession of exercises: rolling, crawling, walking, running, tumbling, falling, climbing over and onto objects, continually picking herself up and doing it again. Just like my young friends at the grammar school!

Upon further reflection I began to see that just as my idea of exercise was very formal and adultlike, so were my ideas about eating, sleeping, eliminating, relaxing, bathing, and nearly everything else I did in daily life. I suppose this should not have come as such a surprise. After all, I was an adult! I ate like an adult was supposed to eat, kept adult-type sleeping hours, did adult-type work, traveled in an adult-type manner. Most of my activities were determined by such adult-like inventions as clocks, calendars, telephones, and automobiles.

The only thing wrong with all this was that I often found myself working when I felt like napping, hungry after eating, and tense after doing something that was supposed to be re-laxing. I had read dozens of books on health, tried several different diets, attended seminars on relaxation, and spent count-less dollars on medicines and doctors for my occasional ailments and aches and pains. The problem was not lack of information. If anything, I suffered from too much. What I wanted was something simple, something that I enjoyed, something that worked.

Curious as to just how much I had changed over the years,

I dusted off a shoebox of old photographs and looked at myself in "the olden days." Memories of lazy, carefree moments floated through my mind: swimming at the beach, building a fort, canoeing at Scout camp, having birthday parties and picnics, camping in my backyard tent. Though the pictures and expressions were an accurate representation of what I had looked like, there was something even more revealing, something that went far beyond the skinny frame, dark skin, close-cropped hair, and ever-present grin. I saw it especially in the eyes. It was a kind of youthful glint — a carefree, rather reckless look that spoke of butterflies and secret forts, marbles in the dirt, supple limbs not afraid to hang from the branches of tall trees.

I put down the pictures and went over to look at myself in the mirror. What I saw was a pale, worried-looking person with a tense jaw, a receding hairline, and a smile punctuated by silver and gold fillings. The eyes were still gray-green and slightly mischievous, but the sparkle was gone. In its place I saw a serious adult, one harried by too many phone calls, appointments, and traffic jams; the glow of childhood had been replaced by the glint of respectability and responsibility.

What had happened? Where was that youthful, carefree lad with the ever-present grin? Where was the boy who ate when he was hungry and slept when he was tired? Was he gone forever, relegated to living in an old shoebox with only occasional outings? Not that I envied his full head of hair and gleaming teeth, or even his skinny legs and waist. I had long since given up worshiping the physical aspects of youth. What attracted me was something more — it was his attitude, his relaxed grin, his confident smile. He seemed to know he could conquer the world. I wasn't so sure anymore.

Over the next few weeks I kept looking at the old photographs. On several afternoons I found myself wandering near the schoolyard; though I did not go in, I felt great pleasure just watching my young friends enjoy recess with such recklessness, such abandon. Somehow it gave me hope. Why, just a few weeks ago I had been one of them!

After giving this matter considerable thought, and allowing for a certain amount of overenthusiasm and dreaminess on the part of an aging adult, I decided that what I really wanted was to be more childlike — but in an adult sort of way. I wanted to find childlike activities I could integrate into my normal adult life — from exercise to food, relaxation to bathing, laughter to tears.

For the next ten years I studied children. I played hide and go seek and hopscotch, climbed trees, and learned to stand on my hands. I observed the way they napped in daytime, the position of their little bodies as they slept at night, their posture, their eating habits, the way they bathed, battled, and breathed. Most of all, I observed their spontaneity, their esprit, their seemingly inexhaustible willingness to take risks and to accept and enjoy life.

And, to the best of my ability, I tried to imitate them. It was not always easy; I was older, more rigid and set in my ways. But I learned, or rather relearned, and the changes I began to feel were familiar. Like the old photographs, the youthfulness I rediscovered was my very own, concealed through decades of unintended neglect, ignorance, and, sometimes, fear. Fortunately, children are patient teachers; they tolerated and helped me while I joined them in their games; they cooperated when I strapped pedometers to their legs to see how many miles they traveled during the day.

Recognizing that children, like adults, have plenty of problems and shortcomings, I took what I considered their most positive and healthy attributes and translated them into activities for adults. The result is a program that is simple, fun, easy to learn, and costs nothing. It requires no special equipment, experience, or advance preparation. If you can yawn and enjoy a good nap, then this program will work for you!

The response has been most gratifying. Through lectures, writing, and the enthusiastic missionary work of many hundreds of reborn children, thousands of people, of all ages and dispositions, have rediscovered not only youthful activities but youthful good health. Like me, they have learned that by making certain simple routines of childhood a part of daily adult life, they can give up such boring activities as exercise and dieting and devote their full attention to what they do best — living.

This book invites you to let childhood bubble to the surface once again. If you're wondering how healthy and childlike you really are, take the Rate Yourself Health Quiz beginning on page 123.

Then take the medicines as prescribed in the chapters of this book. You'll find them sweet and painless, filled with that old-fashioned tonic and elixir — common sense.

Common sense, -sense, 1535 [repr. Gr.] 1. An internal sense which was regarded as the common bond or centre of the five senses 1543. 2. Ordinary, normal, or average understanding (Without this a man is foolish or insane.) 1535. b. Good sound practical sense; general sagacity.

– *The Oxford Universal Dictionary*

✳Following this symbol throughout the book are tips for achieving the success and joy of good health.

Foreword to the 1990 Edition

Twenty years have passed since I first began work on this book — years in which my ideas about health have been altered by dramatic changes in the world around me. When I wrote the chapter on sunlight, for example, I urged people to spend more time outdoors, in the open air. Now, with reported damage to the earth's ozone layer and an alarming increase in skin cancer, I must caution readers about the dangers of sun exposure and remind them to use protective clothing and sunscreen. Twenty years ago I urged readers to do more outdoor aerobic activity, particularly brisk walking. Today the same advice followed in an urban, industrial area could expose people to increased levels of airborne toxins. Water, too, has become increasingly polluted, and water quality is one of our great public concerns.

The magnitude of our environmental problems has left people stunned and frightened. Many have responded by trying to shut the problems out of their minds, hoping that they will somehow go away, that nature will heal itself or that technology will discover something to clean up the air and water, mend the ozone layer, and cure cancer. Is this realistic? And if it isn't, how do we deal with our problems? How can we save our forests and still read the Sunday paper? How can we refrigerate our food and still protect the ozone layer? How can we drive our cars and keep the air clean? In short, how can we preserve the earth and continue to enjoy its gifts?

An old Bedouin proverb says, "Trust in god but tie your camel." What it means is this: even as we pray and wish for a better world, we must also get busy and work to make it happen. Just as personal health can only be realized by the daily practice of simple health disciplines, global health can only be achieved through simple daily efforts.

The quiet efforts of one woman, now in her seventies, well illustrate this point. Each morning she goes for a brisk walk in her neighborhood, and as she walks she stops from time to time to pick up litter — a bottle, a scrap of paper, a plastic cup. The first time I met her I found her litter-collecting stops an annoyance; they broke up the cadence of my aerobic walking. But she was so adept at the collecting, scooping up litter and just barely breaking stride, and she seemed to be having such a good time doing it, that I soon started picking up a few pieces of litter myself. Over the years this woman, without fanfare or attempts to convert others, has motivated many people, myself included, to pick up litter — and has made the streets of our community more beautiful.

This simple principle of human behavior is often overlooked. We think the task is too large for us to do alone, or we wait for someone else to take the initiative. We forget that, like children, we learn by imitation, and that everything we do — every small act — is witnessed and ultimately copied. The magnitude of the act is not important. The regularity is. It is like saving: a few coins put aside each day will, over time, become a significant amount. Healthy people continually find areas in which small tasks, done regularly, help improve the quality of human life.

Despite depressing news via television, radio, and newspapers, a great number of positive things are happening in the world each day. For every destructive act reported, thousands of constructive acts go unreported. For every failure there are thousands of successes. For every misfortune there are thousands of good fortunes. In short, there are always far more things right with the world than there are wrong. Similarly, the health and vitality of each individual far outweighs his or her deficiencies and illnesses. This is important. Instead of treating illness, we can more profitably spend our time promoting health. Instead of dwelling on the problems that confront society, we can better use our time improving the communities in which we live. This approach yields great results. People who learn to appreciate and utilize their strengths soon find their weaknesses diminishing in importance. In the same way, the ailments of society cannot thrive when people apply themselves to simple, creative solutions.

The following story says it best. Frank, a service station attendant, was gloomy for several months. He was working long hours and feeling generally unappreciated by both his boss and his busy customers. One day, when Frank was feeling especially despondent, he received a postcard from an anonymous customer, thanking him for the conscientious way in which he had cleaned a car's windshield. He was so pleased with this unexpected compliment — the first he had received in months — that he read the card several times, showed it to all his colleagues and friends, and posted it in a prominent place, where he would be sure to see it every day. After that Frank's disposition improved steadily. One day, acting on an impulse, he sent a postcard himself — to the mayor of the city. In this card he congratulated the mayor for his efforts to improve public transportation and expressed his concern about the lack of playgrounds for his children. To his surprise, Frank received a reply inviting him to join a volunteer citizen committee working to improve public parks. Frank accepted and thus began a new and exciting life as an involved member of his community.

This book has one simple objective: to inspire you, dear

reader, to improve your own health and that of the earth we share. It is my sincere hope that you will take the renewed vitality that results from following these prescriptions and turn it speedily and enthusiastically toward the betterment of society.

A portion of the proceeds from sales of this book supports the work of The Nature Conservancy. Information on The Nature Conservancy can be found on page 179.

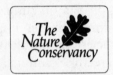

The Art of
Good Living

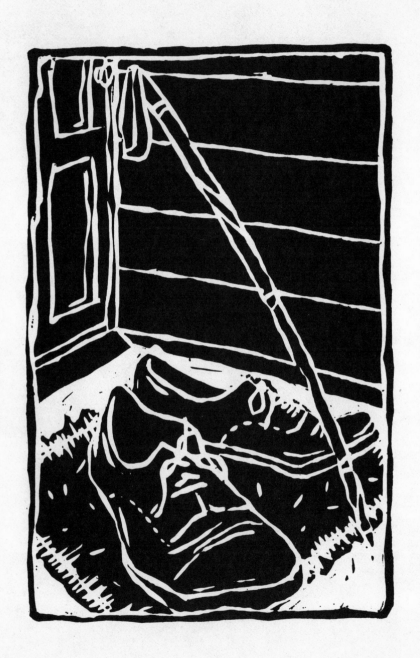

Chapter 1

℞: Child's Play and Vitamin O

THE HEALTHY human organism is a truly remarkable instrument. It can climb trees, jump over ditches, crawl under bushes, swim across rivers, and walk or run for miles and miles without stopping. Of course, after all this exertion, it often collapses in a heap and goes to sleep. But after a few hours' rest and something to eat, it wakes up and is ready to do it all over again!

Given this incredible vitality and range of movement, why is it that after a few years, sometimes only two or three decades, a simple task like climbing a ladder, bending, or lifting a box can become difficult and even painful? Why is it that we begin to wake up stiff and that climbing a flight of stairs can take our breath away? Why does the young body that crouches, jumps, hangs, runs, and twists with such ease and grace become unresponsive, a body full of pain and frustration?

Many people feel the aging process itself is a villain. Aches and pains are part of growing older, they assert, and no amount of wishful thinking can change that. Then, too, it is often argued that most physical disabilities and liabilities are passed along within the family, a kind of genetic predisposition: we are stuck with whatever fortune of health we have brought into the world.

Are these arguments valid? Must we simply roll over and accept ill health because we are getting older or because our parents were ailing? While acknowledging that heredity and age influence health, studies in recent years show conclusively that age and heredity are not the major determinants of health. In fact, the single most important thing that determines our health is attitude. That is, if we believe there is nothing we can do to shake off deteriorating health, chances are nothing will be done. On the other hand, those who feel they can do something, and then do it, witness substantial improvements in their health. In short, our health is as vibrant as we allow it to be.

Still, the question persists: why the deterioration? If age and heredity are not responsible, what is? And what can we do about it?

One of the most important explanations is surely our sedentary existence. Most of us have simply gotten lazy: riding in cars instead of walking, using machines instead of our bodies, sitting long hours behind desks and steering wheels and in front of television sets. The exercise involved in gathering food is often no more than the exercise we get pushing a shopping cart down the aisle of the grocery store. Heating our homes, which once required the cutting and carrying of wood, is now accomplished by moving a tiny lever on the thermostat.

Furthermore, even though our daily activities may include some measure of active physical labor, this work, ironically, often contributes to a deterioration of our health. Because so much work is involved, either directly or indirectly, with modern machinery, we are often required to use our bodies and minds in stress-producing ways: straining our eyes to fit tiny parts into machinery; handling substances that are toxic; doing repetitive movements that create uneven wear on one part of the body; sitting in one position for hours at a time; standing long hours on hard surfaces.

Another explanation for our increasing aches and pains is

the fact that society continually encourages us to think it is normal to be overweight, sluggish, stiff, sedentary, constipated, lethargic, and grumpy. Television, radio, newspapers, magazines, and billboards make it extremely attractive to eat more, drive more, and buy more "labor-saving" gadgets so we don't have to move so much. Aspirin, antacids, and laxatives have been so glorified and promoted as panaceas for our ailments that many of us have come to accept as inevitable the headaches, pains, and constipation they purport to cure. There are few commercials encouraging us to walk, bicycle, play, and relax.

This alienation from play and movement is also reinforced by economic considerations. As we become more affluent we are encouraged to use electric washing machines, can openers, knives, lawn mowers, clothes dryers, and elevators as proof of our economic health. Being a success is often economically defined; even though our health has deteriorated, we are considered successful because our financial health is so vibrant.

Many of us, unfortunately, are not aware that there are alternatives to this deterioration. We accept stiff joints, sore backs, headaches, and glasses as "natural at my age." We become experts at making accommodations, slowly eliminating certain movements and activities, telling ourselves, "I'm not as young as I used to be." As a result, many of us enjoy movement mainly as spectators, by watching others on television or in a stadium.

The truth is that most of us have lost our enthusiasm for childlike behavior — and a good deal of the body stamina and flexibility that went with it. And we're not too excited about joining an exercise class or going through a special routine each day to get it back — which is not surprising. Exercise, as we know it today, is often a drudgery; after a few weeks or months we usually find some very good reasons for not doing it anymore.

Fortunately, it is possible to recover the full range of body movement without doing special exercises — even for those who huff and puff at the mere thought of exertion.

Before beginning, however, it is helpful to understand that in order to function harmoniously, the body needs the stimulation of two distinctly different kinds of movement — endurance and stretching.

Endurance and Stretching

Endurance movements are necessary to build stamina and to increase oxygen intake and the capacity to use that oxygen. These movements, such as walking, running, bicycling, and swimming for long distances, strengthen the heart and respiratory system. They are discussed in the second part of this chapter.

Stretching movements are necessary to keep the body supple and limber, able to bend, twist, squat, and move with ease. These movements prevent stiffness and muscular discomfort. They help keep the spine flexible and healthy. These are the playful stretches of young children and the supple movements of those who do simple manual labor that requires a great variety of body postures.

Although there are many good stretching techniques,* it has been my experience over the years that the very best program is one that is simple, fun, and takes very little time. The program suggested here is just that: it is enjoyable, takes only six minutes a day, and is so simple a baby can do it — which is not surprising, since these are natural movements that babies and children do every day.

---

* For a complete program of stretching movements, see "General Flexibility," Appendix B, page 146.

CHILD'S PLAY AND VITAMIN O

NATURAL STRETCHING MOVEMENTS

1. Yawning

Here is a gentle stretch used by a famous mime as a limbering-up movement prior to performances. I have prescribed it for myself and my patients for many years — to wake up in the morning, to get out the kinks while sitting at a desk, or just to stretch and relax during the day or before bed. If you like, try it right now — it may be a welcome respite from all this sedentary reading.

This may be done while standing, sitting, or even while lying in bed.

Imagine a yawn. Open your mouth as wide as possible and stretch your arms up and away from your body. Move your mouth as though you are really about to yawn. Stretch the jaw muscles. As you reach up, loosen your fingers and spread them as far apart as possible. If you're standing, go up on your tiptoes.

Keep doing this, opening your mouth for a yawn and stretching your arms. Soon your yawns will be bigger and better and will start coming spontaneously, of their own accord.

＊A yawn is essentially an internal stretch of the lungs, accompanied by a stretching of the jaw, the throat, and all the muscles of the face. This spontaneous stretching relieves strain in the eyes, brows, cheeks, and lips. As a result, we are more relaxed and mental tension is relieved. This is important because tension causes stiffness, pain, and impaired movement.

Yawning may well be the most natural of all exercises. The impulse to yawn should never be suppressed. On the contrary, it should be encouraged, and yawning should be practiced as often as possible, stretching the limbs at the same time. When we yawn, sluggish blood is squeezed out of the tissue and is replaced by fresh blood resulting from the internal stretching of the lungs.

Yawning invigorates, energizes, and wakes us up. When we yawn we are actually doing a full body stretch and taking in more oxygen at the same time. This oxygen, as we shall soon see, produces cellular energy. In short, yawning makes us feel better, more supple, and more energized.

2. The Butterfly

1. Stand with good posture. Clasp your hands behind your neck, lacing your fingers.
2. Inhale slowly through your nose, at the same time pulling your elbows back as far as you can, like the wings of a butterfly opening to the morning sun.
3. Now bend slowly forward, exhaling through your nose, bending your elbows, and bringing your chin to your chest. You are a butterfly with folded wings.
4. Begin inhaling again, pulling your elbows open and back until your butterfly wings are fully spread.
5. Repeat twelve times, breathing slowly through your nose, expanding and contracting your chest with each inhalation and exhalation.

Try it with your eyes closed. Soon you will be moving gently and easily, your wings beating to the rhythm of your heart. This is a wonderful way to start the day or to revitalize yourself when you need a burst of fresh energy. It brings fresh blood to the heart and lungs, gets out kinks and cricks from sleep, blows away emotional cobwebs, and breathes new life into tired bodies and minds.

3. Rocking and Rolling

1. Lie on your back on a soft, well-cushioned mat. Raise your knees to your chest and rock gently back and forth. Breathe through your nose. Rock ten to twelve times.

2. With your knees to your chest, start gently rolling side to side. Use your momentum to help push you off the mat and back toward the opposite side. Roll ten to twelve times.
3. For best results, rock and roll twice a day.
Note: Many people who practice this simple stretch become so enthused they begin doing somersaults — frontward, and even backward!

That's all there is to it. The Magic Three. Done twice daily they take only five or six minutes.

Learning something new is greatly facilitated by two things: observation and imitation. Observation heightens our awareness of what is going on around us — we see what older people are doing and learn from their fortunes and misfortunes. Imitation is how we ultimately learn; by choosing good models and copying them, we learn quickly and thoroughly from the very best teachers.

Observing the movements of animals, children, and other people, for example, is a good way to learn more about natural, harmonious movement. Watch a cat at rest, climbing stairs, sleeping, stalking, eating, resting. In each position it is using its body in a total, dynamic way: there is a constant, flowing redistribution of weight and energy.

Become aware of the way other people use and move their bodies. Watch a youngster breathe, eat, sit, and climb. Observe the way different bodies execute simple and complex movements: lifting, pulling, pounding, relaxing. Become an observer and a student of movement.

Observe yourself. Become aware of how you are using your own body. Do you favor one side to the exclusion of the other? Is this one-sidedness contributing to poor posture and muscular imbalance? Is your body responsive? Does it help you with your daily tasks, and without complaining? Mirrors and friends can provide useful feedback. Become aware of the way your body responds when you talk, walk, lift a box or wash dishes, feel tired or upset. ✳Exercise can be anything from doing situps to chewing a piece of bread.

No matter what kind of activity or play we choose — whether it is walking barefoot on a carpet or on a forest floor, watering the garden, wrestling, yawning, or doing the laundry — it should be enjoyable and give us pleasure and satisfaction. This satisfaction is more than just physical, for as the body becomes more supple, more playful, and more relaxed, the mind also becomes more supple, more playful, and more relaxed.

As from the house your mother sees
You playing round the garden trees,
So you may see, if you will look
Through the windows of this book,
Another child, far, far away,
And in another garden, play.
But do not think you can at all,
By knocking on the window, call
That child to hear you. He intent
Is all on his play-business bent.

He does not hear; he will not look,
Nor yet be lured out of this book.
For, long ago, the truth to say,
He has grown up and gone away,
And it is but a child of air
That lingers in the garden there.

— Robert Louis Stevenson
To Any Reader

Let us turn our attention to the second form of activity, endurance movement, and get reacquainted with an old and familiar friend, walking.

Why Walk?

The basic problem confronting every organism on land is how to bring oxygen most efficiently from the environment into the living cells and at the same time expel as much carbon dioxide as possible. This technique is called respiration, or breathing. It is familiar to all of us. It is beyond the power of the will and goes on automatically as long as we are alive. Whether we are asleep or busy with work, respiration continues, in-breaths and out-breaths corresponding to our body's need for oxygen.

This oxygen, which comprises approximately 21 percent of the air we breathe, is the basic fuel needed for the processes of life. There are other fuels, of course, such as water and solid food, but oxygen is unique because it initiates the combustion that produces energy. This energy is derived from the billions of cells that make up the human organism, cells that are continuously dying and being replaced. These energy-producing cells are totally dependent on the ability of the organism to supply them with oxygen. Thus, we see that oxygen is at the very center of the life process.

However, even though oxygen is in the air that surrounds us, it must still be acquired by the application of effort, since without effort no energy can be produced. This effort must be continuous because the air in the lungs is constantly being used up. The average-size person takes in between ten and seventeen pints of air every minute, in twelve to twenty breaths. This is the amount of air intake at rest, during normal breathing. If we go for a leisurely walk, the air intake increases to approximately twenty-six pints per minute. On a long, playful run or a long, vigorous walk, oxygen intake increases to seventy pints of air or more per minute. This means that the oxygen delivered to the body during exertion is six or seven times what it is when the body is at rest.

Pints of Air per Minute

Rest	10 to 17
Slow walk	26
Vigorous walk	70 plus

Why Oxygen?

The oxygen needed to build healthy cells and produce energy for a vibrant life cannot be produced by normal, at-rest respiration, nor can it be supplied by taking a leisurely walk, or even by short periods of exertion. These activities simply do not deliver enough oxygen to the body. Furthermore, our sedentary existence has made the acquisition of increased oxygen even more important. Overeating and underexercising have bred larger and heavier organisms. These organisms have more cells, more mass, and thus require more oxygen to survive. When only small quantities of oxygen are delivered to a large, inactive body mass, the danger of cell deterioration is greatly increased as cells reach the point of oxygen starvation. What we commonly call a "heart attack" occurs in reality when a certain part of the heart muscle, through diminished blood supply, starves of oxygen and is therefore unable to function.

Likewise, when the oxygen is inadequate in other vital areas, disturbances severe enough to be life-threatening can result.

The energy needed to deliver this larger amount of oxygen must come from exertion. This energy is produced through the most basic and natural movements of the body — brisk walking, strenuous manual labor with hand tools, such as chopping wood or shoveling, and child's play. It is also produced by running slowly, swimming, bicycling, and jumping rope.

There are two other important factors that play a critical role in proper oxygenation of the body: first, the vigorous activity, be it walking or digging in the garden, must be sustained for at least twenty minutes at a time; and second, the activity needs to be performed at least three times each week — roughly speaking, every other day.

The relationship of oxygen, energy, and endurance is perfectly balanced in the child at play. Children innately understand the need for endurance and increased oxygen intake. From the earliest years they begin this training — running, jumping, bicycling — covering miles and miles every day. Without reading any studies, children automatically fill their little bodies with air, and in so doing, build fresh, vibrant cells; strong, resistant organs; and bodies and minds that bubble with the elixir of life.

In "Keep Away" and other games, children may run three miles every hour, with about two hundred pauses in between. A youngster at play can easily cover ten miles in a day, with several hundred pauses. ✳ This is the classic training of long-distance runners and nontechnological people who live without automobiles or electricity. A healthy child can run and play all day because he is constantly getting oxygen, the fuel necessary for peak performance.

Of course most of us are not prepared to live like this; therefore, we must build resistance through adult-type endurance training and adult-type activities. The following case history illustrates what I mean.

In 1982 a woman came to our clinic for nutritional counseling. Mrs. Z, a slender, rather pale woman of thirty-nine, worked as a letter carrier for the post office. During the initial interview she told us that for the past eight years she had taken nutritional supplements but that the expense was becoming a financial burden on her family. Furthermore, she often felt tired and worn out after only a few hours' work. She showed us a list of thirty-one vitamins and supplements, some of which she took twice a day. "It comes to over seventy-eight dollars every month," she said, "but I guess it's worth it. If I quit taking them I feel even worse. But it's making things difficult between me and my husband. He says it's all baloney. He eats exactly what I eat, doesn't take supplements or vitamins, and is *never* sick!"

We gave Mrs. Z a food-activity chart on which she was to record everything she ate and drank for six days, as well as all physical activity. She was to fill in the chart and return in ten days for evaluation.

During the second visit, we learned that Mrs. Z's husband was also a letter carrier, working a rural route where mail delivery was done on foot. Mrs. Z, on the other hand, worked at the central post office and made her deliveries from a small postal jeep, delivering the mail through the window of her vehicle. The activity part of her chart indicated that she was a very sedentary person.

Mrs. Z's food chart showed us that she ate a relatively well-balanced diet. The vitamin and mineral supplements, however, were not sufficient to keep her in good health. We told her this.

"You mean I need still *more* vitamins?" she asked with alarm.

"Yes, indeed," we told her. "You have a vitamin deficiency. You have all the necessary vitamins and minerals — except for one, Vitamin O."

"Vitamin O? I never heard of it."

We explained to Mrs. Z that Vitamin O was not available from food — whether you bought it in the grocery store or grew it yourself. Nor did it come in pill form. The only way she could get it was by walking every day, the way her husband did while delivering mail.

Mrs. Z looked skeptical: she had come to us for nutritional counseling. "What does walking have to do with nutrition?" she asked.

"It's simple. When you walk you get oxygen, which is what we call Vitamin O. That's probably the major difference in diet between you and your husband. He gets a liberal dose of Vitamin O every day, because he walks so much. Follow the walking program we prescribe, take the Vitamin O in daily doses, and you can start cutting down on the supplements you take. It will save you money."

Although Mrs. Z confided that she had her doubts, she nonetheless agreed to try the program, hoping it would reduce their debts and perhaps bring more harmony to the family. We prescribed a vigorous fifteen-minute walk, to be taken every morning. We also told Mrs. Z that as she finished each bottle of vitamins or supplements, she was not to refill it.

Four weeks later we saw Mrs. Z again. She had been following the walking program as prescribed and was making good progress. She said that her husband was very pleased that the monthly bills were being reduced. Tension between them had also been reduced. We told Mrs. Z to increase the length of her walks gradually until she could walk for a half-hour, briskly, without stopping.

Mrs. Z said this wouldn't be any problem. "I probably won't need a special program much longer," she said. "I've put in for a transfer, to the same rural postal station where my husband works. I expect to be walking two or three hours a day — and getting paid for it!"

Later that year we received a letter from Mrs. Z. She told us how much she enjoyed her new job and that she felt livelier and more energetic than she had in years. Her relationship with her husband had greatly improved. She also said that many of her old friends had asked her how she had suddenly become so full of zest and vitality. She told them it was due to a new wonder drug she was taking — "Vitamin O."

Breathing exercises, short bursts of strenuous activity, and even most sports do not provide enough oxygen. Some exercises, such as weightlifting and sprinting, actually produce oxygen debts by using oxygen faster than the organism can supply it. Golf, bowling, and an occasional swim at the beach are not movements that build true endurance and fill the body with fresh oxygen. Only by increasing the amount of oxygen we take in, for sustained periods of time and on a regular basis, can we provide the magic ingredient needed to promote vibrant life.*

Walking is economical. You need only supply the remarkable human machine with a modest amount of good fuel — food, water, air, and love — and it will run for hours, usually without complaining.

Walking is also safe and dependable. Assuming we are in reasonably good health — and look both ways before crossing streets — we can walk hundreds or thousands of miles without repairing or replacing our parts. In fact, walking, if done regularly and vigorously, actually strengthens our machinery: it continually lubricates, tunes, and overhauls our parts, keeping them in good working order.

Walking is surely one of life's greatest pleasures. From our first hesitant steps to our last, we move through life, both literally and figuratively, by placing one foot in front of the other. And though we stub our toes, stumble, and occasionally fall down, we invariably pick ourselves up again and take another step. Despite the convenience of other modes of travel, the human body remains the most perfectly constructed machine for traveling across the earth. Even after journeying in another manner — by horse, train, ship, balloon, plane, automobile, or piggyback — we still feel the unique and unmatched joy of touching down to earth. Our feet, no matter how tired, invariably rejoice as they once again begin transporting us on our journeys through life.

Begin walking anytime. Begin today. Begin right now. After

* A graded program in vigorous walking, similar to the one followed by Mrs. Z, is found in Appendix B, page 152.

reading this chapter, put down the book and go for a walk. Go visit a friend or walk to the store. Take a walk to the nearest park and enjoy the birds and small children who are also enjoying the movement. Walk tall. Throw out your chest and take long, vigorous strides, leading with your hips. Breathe deeply into your abdomen. If you like, whistle or sing as you move along. Enjoy yourself. Forget about how long it is taking. Forget about your job, your bills, your problems. Stop occasionally to smell a flower or pet a dog. When you are tired, slow down or stop and rest.

You think you know all about walking — don't you, now? Well, how do you suppose your lower limbs are held to your body? They are sucked up by two cupping vessels, ("cotyloid" — cup-like cavities,) and held there as long as you live, and longer. At any rate, you think you move them backward and forward at such a rate as your will determines, don't you? On the contrary, they swing just as any other pendulums swing, at a fixed rate, determined by their length. You can alter this by muscular power, as you can take hold of the pendulum of a clock and make it move faster or slower; but your ordinary gait is timed by the same mechanism as the movements of the solar system.

•

I do not deny the attraction of walking. I have bored this ancient city through and through in my daily travels, until I know it as an old inhabitant of a Cheshire knows his cheese. Why, it was I who, in the course of these rambles, discovered that remarkable avenue called Myrtle Street, stretching in one long line from east of the Reservoir to a precipitous and rudely paved cliff which looks down on the grim abode of Science, and beyond it to the far hills; a promenade so delicious in its repose, so cheerfully varied with glimpses down the northern slope into busy Cambridge Street, with its iron river of the horse-railroad, and wheeled barges sliding backward and forward over it — so delightfully closing at its western extremity in sunny courts and passages where I know peace, and beauty, and virtue, and serene old age must be perpetual tenants — so alluring to all who desire to take their daily stroll, in the words of Dr. Watts — "alike unknowing and unknown," — that nothing but a sense of duty would have prompted me to reveal the secret of its existence. I concede, therefore, that walking is an immeasurably fine invention, of which old age ought constantly to avail itself. . . .

•

The pleasure of exercise is due first to a purely physical impression, and secondly to a sense of power in action. The first source of pleasure varies of course with our condition and the state of the surrounding circumstances; the second with the amount and kind of power, and the extent and kind of action. In all forms of active exercise there are three powers simultaneously in action — the will, the muscles, and the intellect. Each of these predominates in different kinds of exercise. In walking, the will and muscles are so accustomed to work together and perform their task with so little expenditure of force, that the intellect is left comparatively free. The mental pleasure of walking, as such, is in the sense of power over all our moving machinery.

–Oliver Wendell Holmes
The Autocrat of the Breakfast Table

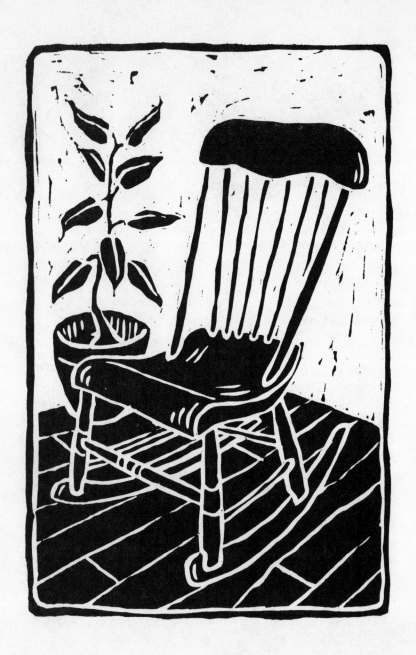

Chapter 2

℞: On the Seventh Day

THE SABBATH, once an integral part of daily life, was designed to guarantee both the earth and its toilers a measure of repose; fields were left fallow so they could recover their tilth; trees were given a "sabbatical" year when fruit was allowed to fall and rot on the ground, thereby renewing the soil beneath them; laborers were granted a day of rest, free from concerns of work and monetary gain.

The idea of the sabbath was well conceived. At a time when nearly everything was done by hand, the importance of rest was understood and appreciated; for upon the quality of rest depended the quality of work that preceded and followed it.

Today, of course, with the proliferation of mechanized labor, demands on the human body are considerably different. The body that once labored in the fields is more likely to be engaged in operating, repairing, and maintaining machinery that works the fields, or calculating profits and losses that accrue from such work. The body that previously harvested fruit from trees is more likely to be doing intellectual tasks that earn money which can be used to purchase this fruit. Toil, in short, is becoming more and more an exercise of the mind; the intricately entwined wires that make up our nervous system and carry the current of life around our bodies are increasingly filled with numbers, figures, facts, and ideas. It is the mind that carries and wields tools. It is the mind that weighs and measures, the mind that toils.

As discussed in Chapter 1, the human organism needs and demands a strong measure of physical activity. Yet, at the same time, this organism needs and demands a strong measure of rest. It is a law of equilibrium and equanimity: for every push there is a pull; for every oomph there must be a corresponding sigh. Just as the honeybee stops her toil each afternoon and takes a short nap in the hive, so too must the human honeybee pause from time to time to rejuvenate and recuperate. And even to rejoice!

Unfortunately, this basic biological need for rest is seldom met. Rather than slowing down, we seem to be going ever faster. Rather than pausing to reflect, we seem to be always accelerating, pushing our bodies and machines toward ever more output and performance. Our appetite for speed and information seems insatiable; we are constantly encouraged to ingest as much of life as we can — in the shortest possible time. In short, we are so busy gathering "human honey" that we rarely take time to rest adequately, to really enjoy the fruits of an intellectual and physical sabbath.

As a result, our nervous systems gradually become strained and overloaded, overstimulated and overextended. After months and years of incessant intellectual activity, often combined with decreased physical activity, the deterioration begins to show: we feel tired; our neck is stiff; we have to strain to move our bowels; we are easily irritated; we spend more time worrying. When we do take time to rest, it is often ineffectual and frequently interrupted; the phone rings or someone asks us to do something. Many times our mind is so full of worries and problems that even though we do stop we are unable truly to rest; our body has stopped but our mind is racing as fast as ever. We begin to get old while we are still young, aging not from the slow, natural wearing away of our wings but from the accelerated deterioration of our nerves.

It has not always been this way. As children, each of us knew how to relax, and we took time to relax. We could lie down in the middle of a roomful of noisy people and go instantly to sleep.

But now that we have grown up, relaxation, or the idea of a sabbath for body and mind, has become a luxury many of us feel we cannot afford. It seems there are never quite enough hours in the day, and if we sneak off and take a nap when there is work to do we feel guilty. Besides, no employer is going to keep us around long if we take off our shoes and close our eyes in the middle of a busy afternoon!

In an attempt to do something about this, we try to relax on weekends or after work. We read, watch television, go for a drive in the country, or play golf or tennis. But these activities, though a welcome relief from our usual routines, demand attention and concentration and are themselves often fatiguing.

Reading, television, and driving, for example, are sedentary activities. They make strong demands on our eyes, keep us relatively immobile, and require a considerable amount of concentration. And sports such as golf and tennis, while beneficial because they include some measure of movement, are competitive and often require intense concentration. Furthermore, we often have to expend a lot of energy just to make this relaxation possible, hurrying to get to the place of relaxation and earning more money so we can afford to relax.

Relaxing and relaxation are frequently confused. Relaxing is the feeling we get while *doing* something. Reading, watching television, driving in the country, and playing golf and tennis are relaxing: they make us feel better; they bring us enjoyment; they are often a nice change from our normal activities. But they do not qualify as rest. We do not come away

from these activities rejuvenated as though we have had a sabbath or a peaceful nap.

* Relaxation, on the other hand, is the feeling we get while
not doing something. It is a resting state, a time when we are
doing nothing. After a period of true relaxation we feel refreshed and invigorated, the way we do after a pleasant nap.

To understand better the distinction between relaxing and
relaxation, let us consider again the delicate balance that exists
in all life.

Listen, for a moment, to your own heartbeat. You will hear
in your pulse the alternate contraction and relaxation of your
heart as it pumps, rests, pumps, rests, pumps, rests.

Similarly, the beat of music and the ebb and flow of waves
in the ocean both contain the same alteration of contraction
and relaxation: the upbeat and downbeat of your foot tapping
to music, and the waves at the beach, followed and preceded
by calm.

Sit at a table. Place your left hand underneath the table,
palm up, and push upward against it. While doing this, use
your right hand to feel the muscles in your upper arm: the
muscle on top (the biceps) is tense and contracted, while the
muscle underneath (the triceps) is soft and relaxed. Now put
your left palm on top of the table, facing down, and push
against it. Notice how it is the triceps (the muscle underneath)
that now tenses tightly, and the biceps that is soft and relaxed.

* This is the way the body works. When an exertion calls
for certain muscles to tense, other muscles relax. Every exertion is therefore balanced with relaxation.

This harmony of exertion and relaxation is found in all aspects of life. Plants expand and contract, going through periods of intense growth, then pulling back into periods of vir-
tual inactivity. Animals rest peacefully, their breaths slow and
controlled. Suddenly they burst into intense, focused exertion — springing, leaping, and chasing. Almost as quickly they

are again at total rest. Children run, jump, leap, and crawl for hours on end. Then, as if by magic, they are silent, all muscles and feelings relaxed in sleep and total relaxation.

Consider your own life. If you are like most people, you are very good at exertion. From the earliest years you were probably encouraged to "do." But how good are you at "not doing"? Are you able to do nothing, and if so, for how long? Can you, at this very moment, shut your eyes and close out everything for two minutes? Try it. For the next two minutes don't do anything. Don't read, don't worry, don't even move your toe.

Did you do it? Can you? If not, you are not alone. Few of us know how to relax completely. It is not taught in schools, and unless we are particularly sensitive to the exertion/relaxation balance we are not likely to practice this simple art. Relaxation is important. It eases tension and renews us. Relaxation promotes opening and receptivity. Relaxation brings greater flexibility, both of body and of mind. It promotes creativity. Relaxation makes it possible to handle change and to turn every situation to our advantage.

Let us use an example, once again, from personal experience. Once while on a long journey I arrived at my destination late at night, by Greyhound bus. I carried with me five or six large parcels and had mentally planned my trip home from the bus station: there was a city bus that would take me nearly to my doorstep.

When I arrived at the station, I claimed my parcels and went outside to catch the local bus. After waiting about a half-hour, and seeing no sign of a bus in any direction, I asked someone and found out that city buses did not operate on Sunday.

I was tired from the long journey, and this news left me both depressed and irritated. My neck and shoulders started to ache, and I felt the onset of a headache. I began to feel hostility toward the bus company that provided no Sunday service.

I considered and rejected several alternatives, and finally called a friend, whose phone rang endlessly. I telephoned the local taxi company and was told my trip would cost twenty dollars and there would be a forty-five-minute wait. Exhausted from the ordeal of the journey and frustrated by my inability to get home, I decided to give up my efforts temporarily and see what, if anything, would happen by not doing anything.

I put all my packages on the ground and sat down, closed my eyes, and let go of a huge sigh. For the next two or three minutes I shut out everything — the traffic, the street lights, my disappointment and anger. Gradually I felt my pulse slow. My shoulders began to droop and relax. The tension slowly drained out of my body.

In this relaxed state I began to see this situation as an opportunity rather than an obstacle. It was like looking at a half glass of water: I could see it as either half full or half empty. Feeling tense and angry, I could see only the emptiness. Now that I was relaxed and more open, I could see that it was still half full. Possibilities for turning this situation to my pleasure and advantage now presented themselves. The solution was suddenly simple, obvious, and clear.

I jumped up, took my luggage back into the bus terminal, and checked my bags once again. Feeling immensely relieved, I went out of the building and began walking, swinging my arms and legs, doing what I had missed all day on the bus — moving. The evening was beautiful and invigorating; I renewed my love for stars, night sounds, and my own footsteps. A half-hour later I was home and happy. The next day, while on my way to visit a friend, I stopped at the bus station and picked up my parcels.

The ability to relax and let go, to diffuse difficult situations and turn them into opportunities, is an art. And like any other art, it must be learned. Just as we learned to read, we can learn to not read. We learned to worry; we can learn to not worry.

We learned how to tense our muscles; we can learn how to untense our muscles. Relaxation is the empty space before and after "doing." It is the nothingness that defines and makes possible what we do. It is a way of standing in a long line and being grateful for the opportunity not to hurry.

In general, increasing the pace tends to increase the level of tension, while decreasing the rate of activity lowers the level of tension. If you chew gum very fast you will notice your jaw is tense. If you slow down and just barely chew, the jaw muscles are again able to relax. Similarly, we can witness our body and mind responding to speed through the raising and lowering of our pulse. When we are in a hurry — driving fast, for example — our pulse is elevated. When we are relaxed, as after a nap, our pulse is slowed.

Thus we see that tension, both physical and emotional, is related to pace. It therefore follows that to relieve tension, to move toward a place of greater repose, we must reduce the pace. This conscious, disciplined slowing down is the secret to learning the art of relaxation.

The art of relaxation — consciously slowing down and not-doing — must be learned and practiced as a discipline. It requires a commitment, a few minutes every day when we give it our complete attention and energy. This means finding a time when we can totally not-do — no cars, no voices, no television, no reading, no worrying. In short, no stimulation, from either the outside or the inside.

"This is all very fine," you say, "but how can I retreat from children, automobiles, telephones, work, laundry, friends, and all my problems? Even when I sleep I can hear the chatter!"

The answer is that in order to learn to relax, we must first acknowledge the importance of relaxation in our lives. Only when relaxation becomes a priority — when we can admit we need to learn to relax — are we ready to learn to relax. Once relaxation is established as a priority we will find time. It may mean giving up a coffee break, a television program, or even fifteen minutes of sleep, but we will find time. We should remember, too, that it is just this — time and pace — that creates tension in the first place. Finding time is an important first step in learning the art of relaxation.

Did you, for example, close your eyes for two minutes as suggested earlier? It's not too late. You can still try it. This time put your fingertips on your wrist so you can feel your pulse. Close your eyes and count about one hundred and fifty beats of your heart. This will be approximately two minutes. If you prefer, ask a friend to tell you when two minutes have passed. Or you can just close your eyes until you think it's been long enough. Two minutes isn't really very long. You can read later, the book won't fly away. Close your eyes. Relax.

". . . When the intolerable midday heat drove us to seek shelter, he (Kalinych) took us to his apiary, into the very heart of the forest. Kalinych opened a little hut for us, hung with bunches of dry scented herbs, made us comfortable on fresh hay while he himself put a sort of sack over his head, took a knife, a pot, and a smoldering stick, and went off to the apiary to cut us some honeycomb. We washed the warm transparent honey down with spring water and fell asleep to the monotonous buzzing of bees and the garrulous rustling of leaves."

—Ivan Turgenev
A Sportsman's Sketches

*The amount of time we actually spend relaxing does not make much difference. It is how well we relax and how well we can apply this relaxation to the rest of our life that is important.

Some people, for example, spend a lot of time in this state of formal relaxation. They sleep, nap, and meditate — sometimes several hours a day. But the rest of the time, when not formally relaxing, they are nervous wrecks. They are edgy, irritable, impossible to please, and get upset at the least little thing. The only time they are relaxed is when they are officially relaxing.

The object of true relaxation is to relax and remain so all the time, not just a few minutes a day. This must be learned and practiced, just like driving a car or playing the piano. When we first learn the piano scales, for instance, we must repeat the exercises over and over until they are thoroughly familiar. After a while we can do them with our eyes closed: we know exactly where each black key and each white key is located.

The same is true with relaxation. At first we must practice relaxation every day. We actually have to sit down and formally stop. For two minutes, fifteen minutes — whatever length of time we need in order to learn — we must close our eyes and discipline ourselves to do nothing.

After a while, sometimes in a matter of months, doing nothing becomes easier and easier. We learn to close our eyes and very quickly shut everything out; we begin to relax totally, the way we did as children. Some of us will even rediscover the art of falling instantly asleep — anywhere, anytime.

Eventually we start to practice relaxation even when we aren't formally practicing. We begin to use the relaxation technique in our everyday life; opportunities are suddenly everywhere. The car battery goes dead and we use this as an opportunity to take a long, relaxing walk to work. The telephone rings and we decide not to answer it. Instead, we listen to its sound, like a bell that is ringing for our pleasure. Eventually it stops. Nothing is lost; whoever called can call again later.

This is what true relaxation is about — learning to relax all the time, twenty-four hours a day. Whether standing in a long line in the grocery store or looking at the broken remnants of our favorite lamp, we can calmly see the situation and use it to our advantage. In the grocery store we take the opportunity to close our eyes briefly or to meet a new friend who is also standing in line. The broken lamp gives us the opportunity to get another lamp, to practice our mending skills, or to enjoy the room as it is illuminated without this lamp. There are an infinite number of possibilities.

RELAXATION EXERCISES

1. Napping

Find a comfortable place where you can nap undisturbed, even for three or four minutes. Remove shoes and glasses. Loosen your belt. Make yourself yawn a few times (see page 5). Now follow these instructions carefully:

Breathe out through the mouth and in through the nose, feel the tension drain down and leave through your toes.

2. Candlelight

One evening each week try using candlelight instead of customary electric light. Prepare dinner by candlelight, eat by candlelight, do dishes by candlelight, talk by candlelight, get ready for bed by candlelight.

Candlelight is soothing and relaxing, a comfort to the eyes. It slows down and stretches out everything we do. It can teach us to act and even think with more care and deliberation. It is also very romantic.

For a special treat use a beeswax candle. Its soothing golden light will comfort and caress you. Its delicate aroma will fill you with the nectar and serenity of the hive.

3. Rocking Chair

From our earliest beginning, in the womb, the rhythm of gentle rocking has been ingrained in life. Though most of us have outgrown our cradles, there's no reason why we shouldn't still enjoy the relaxing rhythm of gentle rocking.

The rocking chair has lulled most of us at one time or another; it can do it again. Next time you're tired, need to relax, or just want to take a short pleasure snooze, go sit in a rocking chair. Close your eyes, give a gentle push, and let the movement carry you down the river of relaxation.

4. Sweet Sabbath

Designate some portion of each week as your sabbath. If you cannot manage a full day, then set aside one evening, or even a few hours. If possible, it should be the same time each week; in this way you can look forward to its arrival.

During your sabbath make no plans and engage in none of your normal activities. Unplug the phone. Put away projects and papers. Turn off the radio and television. Don't cook, shop, read, spend money, or labor in any of the customary ways.

At first it will not be easy. Most of us are accustomed to activity, and when there is none we get nervous and anxious, waiting for something to happen. There are sure to be interruptions — unexpected guests, the arrival of the mail, the sudden thought of something important you forgot to do. Ignore these distractions and temptations; let them pass quickly through your mind. Instead, do simple, enjoyable things you would not normally do; play with blocks, go for a walk, lie on your back and look up at the clouds or ceiling, tell a story, take a nap. See how much you can enjoy yourself without the stimulation of your normal activities.

This sabbath, whether it lasts an hour or a complete day, will be most welcome — by your body and your mind. After a few weeks you will begin to savor the time, and the anticipation of its arrival will make the normal activity of your week more enjoyable and tolerable. ✳The sabbath itself may bring some surprises. Like many people, you may discover you actually get more done by doing nothing; freed from normal concerns and constraints, the creative juices of the mind flow in all sorts of intriguing and unexpected ways.

All that summer I had worked in a sort of animal content. Autumn had now come, late autumn, with coolness in the evening air. I was plowing in my upper field — not then mine in fact — and it was a soft afternoon with the earth turning up moist and fragrant.

I had been walking the furrows all day long. I had taken note, as though my life depended upon it, of the occasional stones or roots in my field, I made sure of the adjustment of the harness, I drove with peculiar care to save the horses. With such simple details of the work in hand I had found in my joy to occupy my mind. Up to that moment the most important things in the world had seemed a straight furrow and well-turned corners — to me, then, a profound accomplishment.

I cannot well describe it, save by the analogy of an opening door somewhere within the house of my consciousness. I had been in the dark: I seemed to emerge. I had been bound down: I seemed to leap up — and with a marvellous sudden sense of freedom and joy.

I stopped there in my field and looked up. And it was as if I had never looked up before. I discovered another world. It had been there before, for long and long, but I had never seen nor felt it. All discoveries are made in that way: a man finds the new thing, not in nature but in himself.

It was as though, concerned with plow and harness and furrow, I had never known that the world had height or colour or sweet sounds, or that there was *feeling* in a hillside. I forgot myself, or where I was. I stood a long time motionless. My dominant feeling, if I can express it, was of a strange new friendliness, a warmth, as though these hills, this field about me, the woods, had suddenly spoken to me and caressed me. It was as though I had been accepted in membership, as though I was now recognized, after long trial, as belonging here. . . .

As I stood there I was conscious of the cool tang of burning leaves and brush heaps, the lazy smoke of which floated down the long valley and found me in my field, and finally I heard, as though the sounds were then made for the first time, all the vague murmurs of the country side — a cow-bell somewhere in the distance, the creak of a wagon, the blurred evening hum of birds, insects, frogs. So much it means for a man to stop and look up from his task. So I stood, and I looked up and down with a glow and a thrill which I cannot now look back upon without some envy and a little amusement at the very grandness and seriousness of it all. And I said aloud to myself: "I will be as broad as the earth. I will not be limited."

—David Grayson
Adventures in Contentment

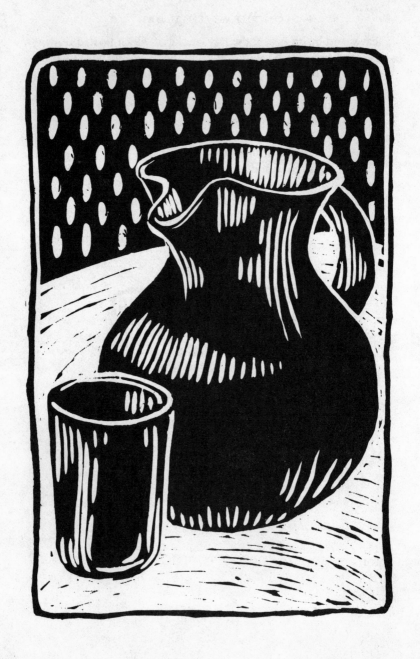

Chapter 3

℞: Turning the Tap

THE TASTE and appreciation for fresh, cool water is generally developed as a child. *Water* is one of the first words we learn to understand and say, and although early attempts to drink often result in overturned glasses and wet floors, water remains a popular beverage and plaything for many years. As we grow older, of course, we learn to appreciate water in many different ways: it washes our clothes, dishes, cars, and pets, nourishes our gardens and plants, and reflects our image when we stare into it. We also come to understand and appreciate water because of the remarkable way it affects our body temperature: when we're cold it warms and soothes us; when we're hot it is cooling and refreshing.

For most of us water is nearly free and nearly always available in unlimited supply. We simply turn the tap and it magically appears. Perhaps this is why we tend to downplay the importance of water, or ignore it completely, favoring instead more glamorous and expensive beverages and medications. We forget that water, when used internally, can be a remarkable restorative of good digestion and elimination, and that when used externally it has the capacity to improve circulation dramatically and bolster resistance to cold and disease. That is what this chapter is about: a gentle yet firm reminder of water's true magic; an understanding of its medicinal and restorative properties and the simple techniques needed to use it wisely and effectively.

First, let us look at the way we relate to water as an internal substance. On a normal day, without exercise or abnormal sweating, nearly two quarts of water leave the body. This takes place mainly through perspiration and kidney and bowel elimination. During strenuous activity, such as manual labor or vigorous exercise, the actual moisture loss can easily be two or three times this amount. Perspiration from sun heat and from nervous sweating further contributes to this loss of moisture.

This means that if the body is to maintain a proper fluid balance, it must take in at least two quarts of water every day. Some of this, of course, comes from our food, but the rest must come from drinking water or water-containing liquids.

Many of us don't drink enough water to maintain a proper, healthy fluid balance; we simply don't replace the moisture lost through normal perspiration and elimination. As a result, our bodies become deprived of fluid. This deprivation, though slow and subtle, contributes to a number of pathological conditions, including sluggishness, headaches, and constipation. ✳ It should be emphasized that most of the time we are not aware of this fluid deficiency and imbalance; we do not feel dehydrated or thirsty, because we have gradually become accustomed to drinking less. Our bodies have also made other subtle accommodations: we tend to sweat less easily, which protects the body from moisture loss but deprives it of the much-needed opening of the pores; our bodies also respond to moisture deficiency by eliminating less frequently.

There are easily understood reasons for the existence of fluid deficiencies. Our increasingly sedentary existence, for example, does not regularly promote sweating. And there are so many "tastier" beverages, such as soda pop, beer, wine, and coffee, which have become much more popular than water. These liquids, however, though largely made up of water, contain other substances — salt, sugar, caffeine, alcohol, etc. — which make them less utilizable and healthful as body fluid.

Still, despite the attraction of other beverages, we have not entirely lost our taste for simple water. Water tumbling down the side of a mountain, for instance, remains one of nature's most divine substances, filled with sunshine, oxygen, and a fragrance and taste that no animal or person can long resist. Under these conditions we marvel at its taste and color, smack our lips with delight, and bottle some to take home.

Meanwhile, back in the city, water as a liquid to drink is not so interesting. After passing through pipes and purifying units, being radiated with antibacterial substances, chlorinated, and sometimes fluoridated, it begins to taste the way it is described in the dictionary: largely odorless, colorless, and tasteless — or even worse. Little wonder that we prefer liquid that has been boiled, salted, sugared, colored, and fermented. The result is obvious: we don't drink as much water as we need to stay healthy, and what we do drink is not water in its natural, fortifying state.

Given the quality of most drinking water and the popularity of other beverages, one can legitimately ask: "Is there a way to improve the taste and quality of water and make it a more interesting drink?"

Fortunately, there are ways to improve ordinary tap water. These techniques are not expensive, nor do they take much time. They require only that you have a sincere interest in improving your health by drinking more water.

First, most water can be greatly improved simply by boiling it. This water can then be cooled, bottled, and drunk whenever you are thirsty. *This is the most ancient and reliable water purification technique; not only are impurities driven from the water, but the taste is markedly improved. For best results, boil the water vigorously for at least a half-hour.

A second water purification technique uses two natural water purifiers found in most kitchens — lemon juice and apple cider vinegar. This works in the following manner: ✳For every quart of water, add one teaspoon apple cider vinegar or lemon juice. Stir and allow to stand overnight or at least eight hours. The resulting liquid is very tasty and may be drunk plain or made into an enjoyable hot drink by warming the water and adding a dab of honey.

The third way to improve ordinary tap water and make it tastier and more nutritious is to make hot tea. This, of course, is familiar, but we do not usually boil the water long enough to really purify it; again, tap water should be boiled vigorously for a half-hour before it is used. Then steep a noncaffeinated tea in the customary manner. Many teas available today will satisfy the palate of even the most confirmed coffee or black tea drinker. Experiment with different teas and blends until you find ones that are satisfying to you. Hibiscus flower tea, for example, is very tasty: in winter it is a bolstering, fortifying drink, in summer a cool, refreshing respite from the heat. It is also a favorite of children when made into delicious red ice pops, and is readily available in most tea shops and supermarkets.

Now, using one of these simple rejuvenation techniques, begin watering your own internal garden. Drink a glass of water when you get up in the morning. Drink another in the evening. Drink several during the day. ✳Increase the amount little by little each week until you are drinking six to eight glasses of water every day. Do not take in great gulps at one time; it is better to drink small quantities a number of times during the day. You will find these delicious drinks to be satisfying and nourishing, a simple way to turn the kitchen faucet into your own private mountain stream. You will once again discover the pleasure of drinking water — the purest, cheapest, and most nourishing tonic and elixir ever concocted.

The second important, yet often overlooked, use of water is as an external wash. Naturally, all of us are familiar with washing in water that has been heated to a pleasingly warm temperature. What has been overlooked is the use of water at lower temperatures, i.e., cool water — water with a temperature below body temperature.

Many readers will be immediately wary of this topic. Some will recoil at the mere thought of cool water touching their skin. Others may already be shivering! Please do not be frightened by the words *cool water*. There is nothing to fear. Cool water bathing has enjoyed a rather sensational reputation, fostered by newspaper photographs showing ninety-year-olds chopping holes in the ice and bathing in the middle of winter. This publicity does cool water bathing a disservice. The truth is that cool water bathing does not involve icy or even very cold water, nor is it limited to health buffs who swim in the ocean in the middle of a cold northern winter. Cool water bathing is actually safe, sane, and "good for ye," as they say. Furthermore, anyone, at any age, can do it right in his or her own home. If approached properly and prudently, cool water bathing is an agreeable experience, any time of year.

The first and most frequently asked question that comes up is "Why bathe in cool water?" — especially when just a few inches away is a tap that can provide one of life's greatest pleasures, a soothing and relaxing hot shower or bath.

Before answering this important question, let me assure you that cool water bathing does not necessitate giving up warm water bathing. In fact, without warm water or some similar heating device, cool water bathing would not be possible — except perhaps for "polar bears," those inimitable old-timers in Chicago and other cities who plunge into the icy waters in midwinter. For the rest of us mortals, cool water and warm water remain close friends; they comfort and moderate each other, thereby maximizing our health and pleasure.

Now, about the benefits of cool water. First, cool water is without a doubt the cheapest and most powerful tonic and constitutional stimulant on the market. There is no drug or elixir quite as powerful.

＊Cool water bathing, if done judiciously and regularly, greatly strengthens the body's defenses. In fact, after a few months of cool water bathing you will begin to notice a greater tolerance for cold air, cold wind, and changes in temperature. You will need less clothing out of doors. You may find yourself opening windows and doors to allow the passage of cool, fresh air into your home or office. You will need less artificial heat to keep your body warm; your own internal thermostat will click on and provide the necessary heat. In short, a cool water rinse is like a breath of fresh air; it clears the cobwebs from the head and gives a welcome burst of vim and vigor.

True, you say, cool water bathing may well awaken a strong instinct for survival. Great-Grandmother herself once said so. But how, after years of bathing in steaming tubs of hot water, can I learn to tolerate cool water? The mere thought of it is chilling.

Cool Water Is Any Water
Below Blood Heat (98.6°F)

It is important to understand that cool water is any water below normal body temperature. When we speak of cool water bathing we are not talking about icy water from the ocean or a mountain stream.

Those of us who could benefit from cool water bathing are often discouraged because we begin by bathing in water that is too cold. The idea is to bathe in cooler water than we are now using. Very gradually we can bathe in progressively cooler water. ＊Remember, any water below blood heat is cold enough to produce the desired benefits previously mentioned.

Cool Water and Healthy Skin

To appreciate fully how cool water bathing affects health, we should also understand how important the skin is to the body. Aside from its role as a protective covering, the skin has several other important functions. By means of the senses of feeling and touch, it conveys sensations to the brain. It is also the regulator of body temperature, functions as an accessory organ of breathing, absorbs substances presented to its surface, and is always busy excreting waste products from the system, mainly through perspiration. To carry on this work, the skin is constantly renewing itself, casting off thousands of old, dead cells every twenty-four hours and replacing them with thousands of new cells which push up from underneath. The scales we can brush off while bathing are actually the dead cells that have been pushed to the surface of the skin.

Healthy skin — skin that eliminates waste efficiently, absorbs, breathes, regulates temperature, and produces new, healthy cells — is promoted by the production of heat internally (sweating through exertion, as discussed in Chapter 1) and exposure of the skin to cool air and cool water externally. When cool water or air touches warm skin it stimulates it, makes it more alive and responsive. ✳ Skin that has been gradually exposed to cool water and cool air over a long period of time becomes strong and resilient, an inhospitable environment for rashes, allergies, and skin irritations.

Cool Water and Warm Sun: The Natural Instinct

The instinct needed to understand and use cool water for bathing is naturally present in every person. It is the same instinct that makes us shiver to produce heat and motivates us

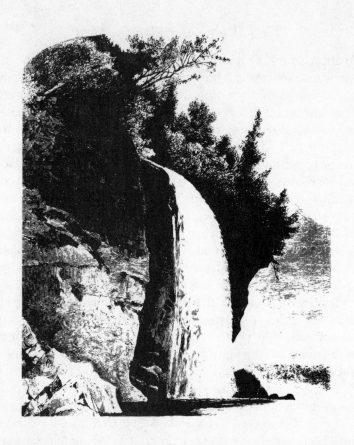

to wear cool clothing on hot summer days. It is the natural reaction of the organism, which inherently seeks balance and equilibrium between hot and cold, between activity and rest.

Consider for a moment what it is like to sunbathe on a warm summer day. You are lying down, perspiring from the hot sun. When you can no longer tolerate the heat, you get up and go into the nearest body of cool water — a swimming pool, a lake, a sprinkler, the ocean, a shower — whatever is available. The water is cool, yet feels deliciously soothing to your warm skin. You get out of the water and begin sunbathing again. Soon you are warm and dry. In a few minutes you are ready to cool off again. ✳ This process, whereby you have gone from warm to cool and then back to warm again, is the basic formula for all cool water bathing.

With this simple formula you can use cool water any time of year, under any conditions. The only rules are (1) that you use cool water only after the body has been sufficiently warmed (otherwise you will chill), (2) that you always finish with cool water, because this closes the pores and protects the body, and (3) that after using cool water, you stay warm by immediately drying and putting on warm clothes, drying in the sun, etc.

These conditions may be met in many ways, of course. In summer you may be able to go directly into a cool shower after working in the yard, and even in winter you may find cool water welcome after a long, vigorous walk. In these situations, where body heat has been generated through exertion, warm water won't be necessary before your cool shower. This is called active heat, because you bring it forth from your own active efforts. It comes from within.

In colder weather, or at times when you are less active, it may be desirable to heat the body in a more passive manner before bathing in cool water. Taking a sauna, standing in front of a fire, sunbathing, lying in a very warm bed, or taking a warm shower or bath may be the preparation needed for cool water bathing. These are examples of passive heat — it comes from the outside and is not generated by the body itself.

Experiment with both active and passive heat production prior to cool water bathing. And keep in mind that active heat, because it requires more energy on your part, is the most beneficial way to heat the body. Each of us, at one time or another, has experienced the release and satisfaction that come from a good workout. We are hot, but happily hot. Our pores open and let out a little bit of what we are. With the perspiration comes a wonderfully satisfying release. Being warmed in this way is the perfect opportunity to enjoy a short splash of cool water.

Turning the Tap

Not many years ago the Saturday night bath was a family institution. Mother, father, children, grandparents, friends, neighbors, and sometimes even family pets would get a good scrubbing in a tub of hot water. This was a ritual everyone looked forward to, except perhaps some of the young ones who didn't see why it was so important to wash behind the ears.

Today, of course, bathing is much simpler. We don't have to gather wood, build a fire, and heat pots of water just to take

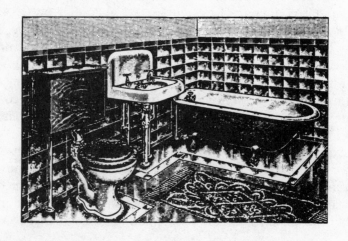

a hot bath. By merely turning the tap (and paying a monthly electric bill!), we enable a virtually unlimited supply of water to cascade from our own private waterfall. And, miraculously enough, we can regulate the waterfall to any temperature we choose. It can be steaming hot like the water from an underground geyser, warm and soothing like the temperature of the blood, cool and refreshing like a gentle breeze, or icy cold like the streams that rush down snow-capped mountains. The choice is ours.

We have the power, by merely turning the tap, to regulate the forces of nature. We should use these forces to our health's greatest advantage.

Some Words of Advice on Cool Water Bathing

✳ A five-second cool shower, taken every day, is far better than one thirty-second cool shower taken only once a week.

Remember that the secret to cool water bathing lies in the reaction of the bather to the water. The desirable reaction may be realized with water only slightly below blood heat. It doesn't have to be icy cold.

Never begin a cool water application if the body is chilled, and never let the body get chilled after using cool water. Cool water is powerful medicine and must be treated with respect. The abuse of cool water — using too much or bathing without adequate preparation — can undermine one's health.

Finish every water application with cool water. ✳ Every time you use hot or warm water — for bathing, shaving, even just washing your hands — finish with a short rinse of cool water. This closes the pores, thus sealing off and protecting the body. Warm water opens the pores. If the pores are left open, the body remains vulnerable to cold.

The entire body should be washed as evenly as possible with

the cool water. This application should feel like a gentle massage.

Brain Wash

Rinse your head with cool water. Massage the water into the scalp with your fingertips. Massage vigorously all over — the back, sides, around the ears — until your head tingles and feels totally alive. A friend's fingers can make this even more enjoyable.

The combination of vigorous massage and cool water on the scalp makes this one of the most delightful and invigorating of all cool water applications. ✳The rush of fresh blood stimulates the scalp and encourages the growth of healthy hair. It also helps keep the hair clean, neither too oily nor too dry.

Sponge Bath

Wet your hands or a sponge with cool water. Then, beginning with the back of the neck, wash your entire body.

Begin with body temperature sponge baths, then gradually use colder water. This is a mild, soothing application, good for those using cool water for the first time. ✳It is also a convenient, refreshing way to bathe when you don't have time for a bath or a shower, and a gentle way to introduce children to cool water bathing.

Foot Bath

Cool water foot baths are a great aid to circulation (especially the veins) and the general improvement of health. As the feet are channels for the nervous and excretory systems, their tone and maintenance are important to the harmonious functioning of the body. Proper bathing of the feet brings them alive. Plunging hot, tired feet into a cool mountain stream or under a faucet of cool water is one of the great pleasures of life.

Skin Brushing

After you finish bathing, with the final cool water application still fresh on the skin, brush your skin vigorously with a firm bristly brush, luffa sponge, sisal mitt, washcloth, or anything slightly abrasive.

This vigorous rubbing of the skin creates friction and heat and if done with enough oomph replaces the need for towel drying or any other means of reheating the body. ✳ Moreover, it removes old, dead skin from the surface of the body, clears the way for good elimination through the pores, and generally brings a nice healthy glow to the skin.

Skin brushing is a wonderful pick-me-up and tonic, one of the best ways to promote healthy, happy skin.

Abstemious in the matter of drinks, the Greeks produce their own light wines and cognacs in abundance. Yet during our whole stay here we have seen a drunk person not more than once; and more endearing still, we have discovered that these people have so delicate a palate as to be connoisseurs of cold water. The glass of water appears everywhere; it is an adjunct to every kind of sweetmeat, and even to alcohol. It has a kind of biblical significance. When a Greek drinks water he *tastes* it, and pressing it against the palate, savours it. The peasants will readily tell you which wells give the sweetest water, and are able to recognize the different sources from which the little white town handcarts (covered in green boughs) are replenished.

Two days before Christmas we climbed the dizzy barren razorback of Pantocratoras to the monastery from which the whole strait lay bare, lazy and dancing in the cold haze. Lines of dazzling water crept out from Butrinto, and southward, like a beetle on a plate, the Italian steamer jogged its six knots towards Ithaca. Clouds were massing over Albania, but the flat lands of Epirus were frosty bright. In the little cell of the warden monk, whose windows gave directly upon the distant sea, and the vague rulings of waves to the east, we sat at a deal table and accepted the most royal of hospitalities — fresh mountain walnuts and pure water from the highest spring; water that had been carried up on the backs of women in stone jars for several hundred feet.

–Lawrence Durrell
Prospero's Cell

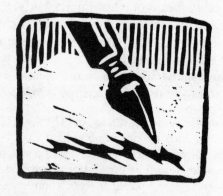

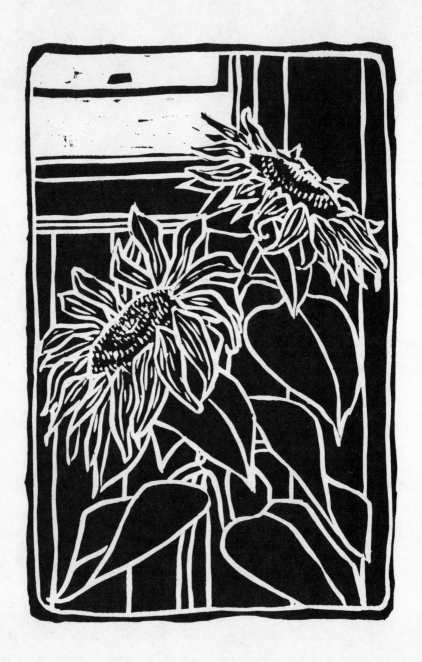

Chapter 4

℞: For the Price
of a Few Clothespins

EVERY DAY the sun's rays wiggle and squirm until they find
us — in homes, cars, factories, schools, and office buildings.
They dart through our clothes, windows, walls, and even our
glasses, in order to caress us. And when they can't touch
us personally, they find other clever ways of doing so: they
shine on cows so the milk we drink is filled with the sun's
warmth and light; they radiate vegetables and fruits as they
grow in fields and orchards so that as we eat them we ingest
the energy of the sun; if we hang our clothes on the line,
they fill them with the sweet nectar of sun so that we may
enjoy their smell and goodness as we wear them. Even on
cloudy, cold days when we can't see or feel the sun's rays,
they are busy doing their work. It is the sun's light, with or
without the sun's heat, that stimulates growth in plants and
animals.

> Great is the sun, and wide he goes
> Through empty heaven without repose;
> And in the blue and glowing days
> More thick than rain he showers his rays

Though closer still the blinds we pull
To keep the shady parlor cool,
Yet he will find a chink or two
To slip his golden fingers through.

—Robert Louis Stevenson

Before taking a closer look at our relationship to the sun, let us see what sunlight actually does to promote good health. First, sunlight has a long and well-deserved reputation as an important nutrient. In warmer months, particularly spring and summer, when we spend more time outdoors, illnesses such as colds and flu occur infrequently and disappear quickly when they do happen. Mothers, in particular, have always recognized the importance of the sun as a nourishing and healthful substance; for thousands of years they have been clearing up their children's runny noses by "dosing" them with the sun's light. It has also been observed and well documented that in winter, when we spend more time indoors, the incidence of colds, flu, anemia, and infections is greatly increased. These "illnesses of darkness," as they are called, are most serious in large cities, where tall buildings shut out sunlight and people are forced to huddle in cars, buildings, and heavy clothing to escape the cold.

Sunlight nourishes the body through contact with the skin, which extracts vitamin D from it. This happens because the skin, the largest organ of the body, is perfectly constructed to absorb sunlight. When exposed regularly to light (not the sun's heat), the skin becomes a supple, vibrant tissue. You can see this quite readily in children who play outdoors every day, no matter what the weather: they have shiny, well-toned skin and glowing cheeks, which only exposure to sunlight, wind, and fresh air can color in such a luxurious manner.

＊Sunlight also influences the chemistry of our blood. Extensive testing has shown that our blood is enriched in iron and phosphorus as exposure to sunlight increases. Recent studies indicate that sunlight helps the body utilize calcium more efficiently. There is no vitamin or tonic, natural or unnatural, that can compare with the blood-building power of sunlight.

Sunlight is also important because of its positive influence on our nervous system. ✳When light bathes our eyes, particularly when unfiltered by eyeglasses and window glass, the entire body is toned and energized. The importance of light contact with the eyes is well known to blind people; it is the light striking the eye that enables them to "see" and feel even though their vision is impaired.

The evidence is mounting that natural sunlight is important to our health. A recent study of college students demonstrated that students exposed regularly to natural sunlight have greater visual acuity than students who are exposed only to artificial light. Several years ago, an International Commission on Illumination was formed to bring together research and information on the effects of light on people and animals around the world.

Given the remarkable gifts the sun bestows on the human body, why does it have such a bad reputation? It is blamed not only for global drought but also for an epidemic of melanoma, or skin cancer. Unfortunately, ignorance about how to use the sun safely, coupled with environmental pollutants that have partially destroyed the earth's ozone layer, has rendered the sun's rays increasingly dangerous. Instead of benefiting from the sun's offerings, many now find themselves suffering sun-related illnesses.

What can we do about this? How can we benefit from the sun's beauty, allure, and remarkable properties without risk to our health? Fortunately, there are ways to improve our relationship with the golden ball that greets us each morning and tucks us into bed each night.

For one thing, we must begin to appreciate the sun for its light as well as its heat. Instead of waiting for the day to get hot, we must do our sunbathing while the air is still relatively cool — in the early hours of the morning and the late afternoon. Even in the middle of winter, when the air is cold and the sky is sometimes covered with dark clouds, the healthful offerings of the sun are available in abundance — provided, of course, we use them in a safe manner. Just as we learned in Chapter 3 to bathe in cool water, so we can learn to bathe in cool sunlight.

Second, we should filter the sun's light before it reaches the skin. Leafy trees, clothing, sunglasses, hats, and sunscreen all help protect sensitive skin from the sun's harmful ultraviolet rays. The wise sun worshipper will take sunbaths between seven and nine A.M. and during the rest of the day enjoy sun filtered through sunscreen and protective clothing. Even models and movie stars, formerly noted for their scanty sunbathing apparel and deep tans, are now being photographed wearing long-sleeved shirts, long skirts, and wide-brimmed hats. Fair skin is once more becoming fashionable.

Finally, we must provide more opportunities for filtered natural sunlight to enter our schools, offices, factories, and homes — places where the sun's light is often shut out by thick walls and has been replaced by artificial light. Let us once more take up outdoor activities — gardening, bicycling, and walking — which allow more intimate contact with natural light. Employees in office buildings should be given the chance to take their coffee breaks in natural sunlight. Roof gardens could become shrines for those seeking better health. Outdoor cafés and restaurants, such as those found along the wide, tree-lined boulevards in Paris and other European cities, could provide more natural light exposure during leisure activities.

Every day, year round, the sun shines upon the earth, inviting us to come out and play in its light. Wearing protective clothing and wide-brimmed hats, we must accept the invitation:

> Meanwhile his golden face around
> He bares to all the garden ground,
> And sheds a warm and glittering look
> Among the ivy's inmost nook
>
> Above the hills, along the blue
> Round the bright air with footing true,
> To please the child, to paint the rose,
> The gardener of the World, he goes.
>
> —Robert Louis Stevenson

Each of us, of course, must establish his or her own relationship with the sun. Some people will continue to enjoy sun mainly through direct exposure. Others may prefer to take in sunlight in less direct ways: by enjoying the sun after it has passed through the foliage of a favorite tree; by tasting fruit that has been allowed to sweeten and ripen slowly in the open air; by eating a bright orange winter squash, a nutritious and tasty reminder of past sunshine.

Once worshipped by primitive people as a god, the sun offers many hidden benefits and opportunities. At a time when fossil fuels are being rapidly depleted, more and more people are looking to the sun as a potential source of energy. Radiation from the sun, harnessed and used safely, may prove a powerful medicine in the treatment of modern-day ailments. The sun is old and wise: more reliable and powerful than an electric light; more invigorating, even on a winter day, than the most sophisticated system of artificial heating; stronger, hotter, and cheaper than an electric clothes dryer. For the price of a piece of rope and a few clothespins, we can once again bring the fresh, invigorating fragrance of sunlight into our homes and lives.

HOW TO TAKE A LIGHT BATH

1. Don't be put off by the weather. A brisk walk during a cold, cloudy day, or even during a rain shower, may yield unexpected benefits and pleasures.
2. Wear clothing made from natural fibers — wool, cotton, silk, linen, and others. This will enable the beneficial light rays to penetrate the skin more easily.
3. If you wear glasses or contact lenses, take them off for a few minutes each day to allow unfiltered light to bathe the eyes.
4. Avoid the sun when it is intensely hot or too high in the sky. Try to catch the early morning sun, when the light is most invigorating.
5. Protect the skin by wearing long-sleeved shirts, long dresses or trousers, sunglasses, sun hats, and so forth.
6. Get in the habit of using a good sunscreen with an SPF (skin protection factor) rating of at least 15. Remember, skin damage can occur with very short sun exposure; even five or ten minutes of strong sun can cause damage. Furthermore, the harmful effects are cumulative over the years.
7. Protect children from too much sun exposure. A child's skin is delicate and sensitive, hence more susceptible to sun damage.
8. Remember that pets and animals need light baths as much as we do. The healthiest milk comes from the healthiest cow.

We had a remarkable sunset one day last November. I was walking in a meadow, the source of a small brook, when the sun at last, just before setting, after a cold gray day, reached a clear stratum in the horizon, and the softest, brightest morning sunlight fell on the dry grass and on the stems of the trees in the opposite horizon and on the leaves of the shrub-oaks in the hillside, while our shadows stretched long over the meadow eastward, as if we were the only motes in its beams.

It was such a light as we could not have imagined a moment before, and the air also was so warm and serene that nothing was wanting to make a paradise of that meadow. When we reflected that this was not a solitary phenomenon, never to happen again, but that it would happen forever and ever an infinite number of evenings, and cheer and reassure the latest child that walked there, it was more glorious still.

The sun sets on some retired meadow, where no house is visible, with all the glory and splendor that it lavishes on cities, and perchance as it has never set before — where there is but a solitary marsh-hawk to have his wings gilded by it, or only a musquash looks out from his cabin, and there is some little black-veined brook in the midst of the marsh, just beginning to meander, winding slowly round a decaying stump. We walked in so pure and bright a light, gilding the withered grass and leaves, so softly and serenely bright, I thought I had never bathed in such a golden flood, without a ripple or a murmur to it. The west side of every wood and rising ground gleamed like the boundary of Elysium, and the sun on our backs seemed like a gentle herdsman driving us home at evening.

So we saunter toward the Holy Land, till one day the sun shall shine more brightly than ever he has done, shall perchance shine into our minds and hearts, and light up our whole lives with a great awakening light, as warm and serene and golden as on a bankside in autumn.

–Henry David Thoreau
Excursions

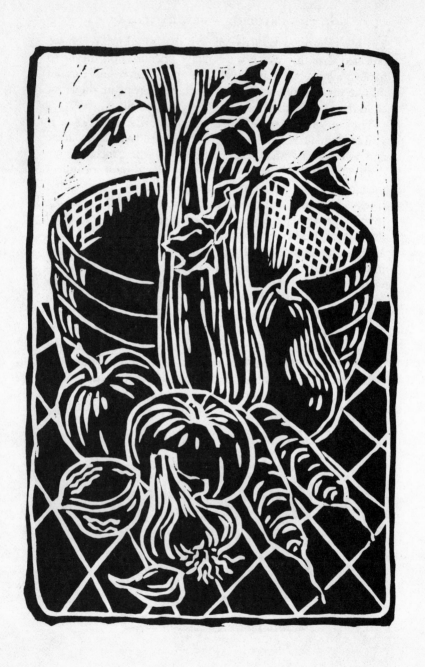

Chapter 5

℞: Diet for a Small, Happy Stomach

IF WE TAKE one hundred people and give them the same fuel — the same air, water, and solids — they will all turn out quite different. Some will be fat, some skinny, some will be happy, some unhappy, some calm, some tense. They will differ in as many ways as it is possible to differ, including size, strength, lifespan, and attitude.

Quite obviously we are what we eat, and a lot more. In fact, one could easily argue that what we do with the fuel — how we assimilate and eliminate it — is even more important than what we put in . A very calm person, for example, will utilize her or his food better than a very tense person. A highly trained person in good health may actually thrive on fuel that renders an untrained and out-of-shape person weak or anemic. And a person with good digestion and efficient elimination may optimally utilize body fuel that causes gas and indigestion in others.

What this means is that in order to talk about food or nutrition, we must also consider such variables as digestion, elimination, and attitude. That is why this chapter dealing with what we put into our bodies is followed by a chapter on what comes out.

Still, food is food, and even though it is not the only factor determining health, we all spend a good portion of our lives gathering it, eating it, earning money to buy it, eliminating it, or just thinking about it. Let us consider for a moment just what a unique and significant role food plays in our lives.

Whereas the other major fuel, air, is largely obtained involuntarily (that is, we breathe without consciously deciding to breathe), our food intake is largely a voluntary act; every time we are hungry or want to eat or drink, we must do something to satisfy that need. When we are babies we nurse or cry until we are fed. As we grow older we begin foraging for food, in fields, gardens, and supermarkets. Even after we gather the food, there are conscious acts involved with using it as fuel: we must prepare it, peel it, wash it, cook it, etc., and then put it in our mouths. ✳This actual picking up of the food with our hands and putting it in our mouths is what makes the food experience so special. It makes our relationship to food both intimate and personal, a relationship that is unique among body fuels.

The problems confronting the person who desires an optimal food experience are first, how to satisfy hunger and cravings for food, and second, how to give the body the food it needs to function optimally.

Satisfaction of hunger is relatively easy, at least for the third of the world that has an overabundance of food: we can grow it ourselves or buy it from those who grow it. The problem is not so much how to appease hunger as how to know when we're really hungry and what to do about it.

Giving our bodies what they need to function optimally is more of a challenge. So many thousands of different foods are readily available every day of the year that making the proper choices has become increasingly difficult.

Take cheese, for example. When we eat cheese we satisfy certain of our body's nutritional requirements, but the dilemma is this: which of the many cheeses for sale at the local market will best meet our nutritional needs? Some are yellow, some red, some white; some are from goats, some from cows; some pasteurized, some homogenized, some raw. Each one, it seems, has been subjected to a different process. And what of the animals from which they come? Are they healthy? Are they fed hormones to increase milk production? Are they kept in pens or allowed to roam in the sunlight? Are they milked by hand or machine? How old is the milk? What effects do the different containers and preservatives have on the milk? On the cheese? Other variables also help determine our relationship with the cheese, ranging from the advertising that accompanies it to the feelings cheese gives us when we eat it.

> The friendly cow all red and white,
> I love with all my heart:
> She gives me cream with all her might,
> To eat with apple-tart.
>
> She wanders lowing here and there,
> And yet she cannot stray,
> All in the pleasant open air,
> The pleasant light of day;
>
> And blown by all the winds that pass
> And wet with all the showers,
> She walks among the meadow grass
> And eats the meadow flowers.
>
> —Robert Louis Stevenson

Considering the amount of food available, it is not surprising that there are so many different theories and philosophies about what we should eat. Nearly every week, it seems, a new diet or food discovery is announced. Special vitamins, cereals laden with protein, and bread boosted with synthetic and natural nutrients all promise to bring us radiant health. The health food industry tells us that only health food can make us healthy. The milk industry says that what we need is more milk. The beef industry says that we should eat more beef. One expert says we can eat anything because food does not affect health. Another expert says our diseases are a result of eating the wrong kinds of foods.

The increased scientific information about food and nutrition has perhaps increased the confusion. Most of us know what proteins, fats, and calories are, yet still don't know how to find a satisfying combination of foods.

There are other factors that make the selection of the right foods difficult and sometimes confusing. A diet that nourishes a farmer in Southeast Asia may be deficient for a farmer in Iowa, a diet that is fortifying for people who live by the sea may be debilitating for people who live in the mountains, and a diet that satisfies the needs of a sedentary person may be inadequate for a person doing hard physical labor. Furthermore, the most nutritious food can have the effect of poison if one is emotionally upset while eating.

Given the many variables involved in the food process, how can we find a diet that is both satisfying and healthful?

As in many other things, the methods that lead to nutritional harmony are deceptively simple. In fact, it is because of their simplicity that they are often overlooked by those seeking more sophisticated paths to better nutrition.

These methods are not new, nor are they difficult to learn. They do not require a special knowledge of nutritional science or how to combine foods; they have been known and practiced for centuries, long before words such as carbohydrates, fats, protein, and calories became a part of our vocabularies.

The only requirement is that you, the reader, study the following information with an open mind, putting aside for the moment all the other ideas you may have accumulated about what constitutes good nutrition. And please do not be deceived by the simplicity of what you are about to read. This simplicity has provided people with healthy, satisfying meals for many centuries. It can do the same for you.

EIGHT PRINCIPLES OF SUPERIOR NUTRITION

1. Eat a Generous Supply of Fresh, Ripe Fruits and Vegetables — Every Day!

The convenience and popularity of prepackaged food has resulted in the gradual disappearance of fresh food from the home. More and more of our food has been sitting in boxes, cans, and freezers for weeks and sometimes even months before we eat it.

There is no substitute for food that is eaten fresh, just as it comes in its own natural package. The tastiest and most nutritious orange juice, for example, is inside the orange itself. It is made by breaking open the orange's container — peeling back the skin — and drinking the fresh juice inside. There is only one brand of orange juice with superior nutritional value — the fresh juice of a real orange. Similarly, nutritionally superior lemonade is made by squeezing a lemon's juice into fresh water and adding a little honey.

Fresh vegetables are also available right in your own kitchen. For just a few pennies a week you can have the satisfaction and nourishment that comes from sprouting grains and seeds such as alfalfa, sunflower,* mung, rye, etc. With a little ingenuity you can turn your home or apartment into a productive little farm, a continuous source of fresh greens for you and your family.

To get the full nutritional value from food, you must eat it when it is thoroughly ripe. ✳Fruits that have not properly

* See "Green Energy," page iii.

ripened are constipating. Fruits that are mature are easily digestible and slightly laxative. Bananas, for example, are not ripe until they are dark and speckled. Avocados when fully ripened are often discarded as being "bad" or "overripe."

✳ Most fruits and vegetables can be ripened by leaving them in sunlight for a few hours prior to eating. This is also a good way to improve the nutritional value of food.

2. Eat Food That Is Whole and Still Has All of Its Edible Components.

Plants, like people, are made up of many different parts. A carrot, for example, has an outer peel and green top in which are stored many important nutrients. If you carefully scrub a carrot with a vegetable brush and make sure its top is free of residue and spray, you can eat the peel and green with the pulp of the carrot itself. ✳ The greens, chopped like parsley, make a tasty addition to salad. When eaten in this manner, with all of its edible components, a carrot becomes a nutritionally complete and superior food. Of course, it is not always possible to eat a carrot like this. Carrot tops are often removed before they reach the market, and strong sprays and chemical residue sometimes make the peeling of carrots (and other fruits and vegetables) a good idea.

Similarly, other foods should be eaten in their entirety whenever possible. Rice, for example, has many of its vitamins and other important elements stored in the hull; therefore, it is important to eat rice in its natural state, with the hull still on. This is usually called brown rice, and has all of its edible components still intact.

So too with seeds and grains. ✳ It is nutritionally important to use them as soon as possible after they have been milled, because in the milling process the grain is crushed open and its contents are exposed to air, with resultant deterioration in nutritional quality. It's no coincidence that bread made from flour that has just been milled from the whole grain is the most delicious and nutritious of all breads.* Bread that is "enriched" is made from grain that has lost its nutritional impact because its edible parts are no longer together the way nature arranged them.

Common Fruits and Vegetables and Their Edible Components: †

Apple:	Eat with peel and some of the core.
Orange:	Eat some of the inner white of the peel.
Grapefruit:	Eat some of the pulp and inner white of the peel.
Pear:	Eat skin and part of the core.
Lemon:	Eat some of the pulp.
Potatoes:	Cook and eat with skins.
Cucumbers:	Eat with peel.
Turnip:	Eat with peel and some of the greens.
Radishes:	Eat with peel and some of the greens.

3. Eat Simpler Meals That Contain Fewer Ingredients yet Deliver More Nutritional Impact.

Eating simpler meals simplifies the entire food process: there are fewer foods to grow and buy, less time is required for food preparation, and there are not so many foods for the body to respond to and digest. If you select these foods with care, concentrating on fresh, raw greens and cooked whole grains, your family will eat better and save money, too. Buckwheat (ka-

* See "Bread and Cooked Whole Grains," page 168.
† Note: Fruits and vegetables that have been sprayed or waxed should be peeled prior to use.

sha),* lima beans, and spinach salad (garnished with apple cider vinegar, olive oil, thyme, and kelp), for example, is easy to prepare and makes a tasty, satisfying, and nutritionally superior meal.

Eating in this manner does not mean less variety of appealing dishes. On the contrary, learning to use a grain in many different ways can be a delightful adventure (see recipes beginning on page 74).

This is not as easy as it sounds, of course. Most of us have become so accustomed to buying and eating whatever we want that it takes time and discipline to eat simpler and fewer kinds of food. It also means we must cruise the supermarkets very carefully, ignoring the thousands of items that are enticing yet have low nutritional value.

At first this may prove to be a hardship for those accustomed to eating a different kind of food at every meal. In time, however, even the most dedicated gourmet will discover the richness of simplicity.

4. Eat According to the Seasons.

Those who observe the rhythm of nature know that each season presents its own bounty of special plants. There are, for example, plants that ripen and mature only when there are long days of hot sun, and others that ripen and mature only in cold weather.

In the warmer months, throughout the summer and early fall, one can eat a procession of beautiful fruits, beginning with pears, apricots, and peaches and ending with autumn apples.

---

*To make buckwheat especially tasty, heat raw hulled buckwheat kernels (called buckwheat groats) in a dry skillet, stirring and turning until they are brown. (You can also start with toasted buckwheat groats. These are more quickly prepared as they need only heating, not browning.) Once the kernels are brown and hot, cover them with hot water and cook for about ten minutes, until they have absorbed the water and become fluffy. The buckwheat will now have an exotic nutty flavor.

This is also a time of abundant fresh greens: peas, lettuce, and onion greens, followed by familiar summer favorites such as cucumbers, tomatoes, green beans, and corn.

These plants, it will be noted, are succulent and juicy, welcome fluid for bodies that have been dehydrated by the sun. Summer is a time for cool beverages, tossed green salads, and fresh, juicy fruits.

As the sun gets lower in the sky, in autumn and winter, different plants flourish. Root crops such as carrots, turnips, and beets are in abundance. Winter fruits such as oranges, lemons, and grapefruits may be obtained quite easily.

Winter is a time of pulling in and contraction. The plants drop their leaves and go into a period of slowed growth. Bees and other insects and animals slow down and go into hibernation, living off the food and fat they have accumulated in the summer months.

In the winter our nutritional needs are different. Concentrated foods such as honey, nuts, dried fruits, and legumes are needed to help produce body heat. Winter is a time for baked potatoes, grains, vegetable oils, and hot soups; a time for eating toast and cheese, and for drinking warm water, lemon, and honey.

Thus, we see that by observing the plants and the seasons, a definite pattern of eating presents itself. It is no accident of nature that citrus fruit ripens in winter, at precisely the time that the body needs those special nutrients, or that nuts that fall from the trees in autumn contain the oils the body needs in the cold of winter.

Below a few common foods are listed according to the season of their maturation. These foods should be eaten frequently and in large quantities in the season when they are available. Eating in this manner will help you eat in a narrower range (see Principle 3) and at the same time in harmony with nature.

It should be noted that some foods, such as cabbage, may

be eaten in several seasons, and that root vegetables, which will keep throughout the winter, may be eaten until the new crops appear in the spring.

Examples of Foods for Warmer Months	*Corresponding Foods for Colder Months*
Fresh corn, beans, peas	Dried corn, beans, peas, cooked whole grains, vegetable oils, nuts and seeds
Garlic and onion greens	Garlic and onion bulbs
Tomatoes, cucumbers, radishes, lettuce, beet and turnip greens	Root crops (turnips, beets, carrots, potatoes), sprouts, cabbage (sauerkraut), kale, squash
Fresh summer fruits (apricots, cherries, pears, melons, peaches, berries, etc.)	Citrus fruits, apples, avocados, winter pears, dried fruit, honey
Milk, yogurt, kefir, soft cheese	Hard cheese

5. Try to Eat 50 Percent or More of Your Food in the Raw, Uncooked State.

Many of us associate raw food with eating an apple or munching on a carrot or a piece of celery. This, unfortunately, is a popular misconception of what it means to eat more raw, unfired food. As we will see in this discussion, raw food preparation is a technique that must be learned and practiced.

In order to eat 50 percent raw food, you must learn the art of preparing appetizing, attractive meals from uncooked foods. It's not hard to learn; all you need is a few simple tools — a grater, a cutting knife, good vegetable oil, a few kitchen herbs, a lemon or apple cider vinegar, and some courage and determination. You will be surprised and delighted at the delicious, attractive meals you can concoct without cooking.

Few of us actually eat 50 percent of our food uncooked. Most cheese, for example, is made from pasteurized milk, which has been heated to a high temperature. Most juices, too, have been pasteurized to prevent deterioration, as in the canning process. When we look more closely at the food substances available, we often discover that somewhere in the packaging or bottling process they have been cooked.

This is unfortunate, because cooking and intense heat leach many important nutrients from food. In general, the longer a vegetable is cooked, the less nutritious it becomes. If, for example, a vegetable is boiled for a half-hour, it loses much of its nutritional value; in this case the discarded water might be more fortifying than the vegetable itself. The point is that many of us are not aware of the great disservice we do ourselves by cooking and overcooking food.

Vegetables that are cooked should be lightly steamed or sauteed and eaten while still crisp. *If it is necessary to cook vegetables in water, be sure to use the water in which they are cooked; either drink it or use it for soup stock.

Soups should be made by warming the broth and adding lightly steamed or sauteed vegetables just before serving. This way the vegetables are crisp and will have retained more of their nutritional value. And don't forget the peels and greens of the vegetables. They are important components of every plant.

Many of the recipes at the end of this chapter have been selected because they can be prepared without cooking. Try a few of them; you will soon learn the simple and satisfying art of raw food preparation.

6. Chew the Food Well.

The way you prepare food for your stomach — how well you chew it — is very important. ✱Even the most nutritious food will not be thoroughly assimilated unless it is properly masticated. The salivary glands are only activated if the food is held in the mouth and thoroughly chewed. The saliva released by these glands helps break down the food and prepare it for its passage through the body. Proper mastication also has other important benefits: by chewing the food longer, you will be satisfied more easily and will eat less, and you will be doing your teeth and gums a favor by letting them do what they were designed to do.

Unfortunately, many of us have lost the habit of chewing. Precooked and convenience foods require very little mastication. They are often washed down quickly with a glass of milk, water, or beer.

Another factor that makes chewing less popular is that it takes more time. Many people consider mealtime something that should be finished as quickly as possible so they can do "more important" things. They don't have the time or patience required to chew their food properly.

It is well known that when people are faced with shortages of food, they quickly learn to take more time chewing; every mouthful is savored and enjoyed, kept in the mouth until well broken down. For those of us who have not experienced food deprivation, it becomes easy to eat and chew quickly, as there is usually plenty more to eat — on the plate, in the refrigerator, at the supermarket.

In the art of proper chewing, it is important to avoid excessive drinking with meals. If there is too much fluid in the mouth, food is washed down too quickly and swallowed in pieces too large for proper digestion. The salivary glands are there to provide all the liquid that is necessary. Chewing is the stimulation these glands need to provide the fluid necessary to start the digestive process.

Many people have successfully learned to masticate their food and eat less by practicing the "Birthday Chew." *This works in the following manner: Every time you eat, choose just one mouthful of food and chew it one time for every year you have been alive. This is a good reminder of how fast we eat and provides a good opportunity to slow down and "ruminate" both food and life.

7. Eat in Moderation.

This is perhaps the most difficult part of better nutrition. Those who do everything else right — eating fresh, whole food daily, eating a narrow range of food, eating according to the seasons, and thoroughly masticating their food — will still have an unsatisfactory food experience if they overeat. The most nourishing food will act like a poison if eaten in excess. Rather than drink a gallon of carrot juice, it might be easier on the system to have a sip of whiskey!

This question is often asked: "What is excess?" Excess, of course, is different for each individual. Most people know when they have eaten enough; there is a little bell that rings and says "full." Many of us, however, have learned to ignore the bells, stretching our stomachs to accommodate ever more food. It has been said that the most difficult exercise of all is pushing away from the dinner table. Even the strongest person in the world finds it a serious challenge.

A few simple techniques can help us learn this difficult exercise.

• Eat from a smaller bowl or plate.
• Take smaller portions of food, filling your bowl several times, if necessary.

- Always leave some food in your plate or bowl when you have finished eating. *Food in the plate or bowl is the signal to stop eating.
- Eat when you are relaxed. Avoid eating while standing, working, lying down, or watching television. Make eating a special experience. Sit down, take your time. Sit up straight. Take a few deep breaths. Put all your energy into the eating experience.
- Avoid eating between meals. If you are hungry, eat fresh fruit or drink tea or water.
- Drink six to eight glasses of fresh water every day. This is a great aid to elimination and helps control the appetite.
- Avoid eating a large meal close to bedtime. When the stomach is full of food, the body must stay busy with digestion. This interferes with total rest. Try eating a larger breakfast and a smaller dinner. This helps many people get through the day without overeating.
- Fasting one day a month or one day a week is an excellent way to accustom both body and mind to eating less. If possible, go without food the same day each week. On this day drink only plain water or water with a few drops of fresh lemon juice or apple cider vinegar. This weekly fast gives the organs of the body a chance to rest. It also provides a sabbath for the mind, which is so often preoccupied with eating.*

8. Exercise Vigorously Three or Four Times a Week.

Many people will ask, "What does exercise have to do with food and eating?" The answer is "Everything."

Those of us who want a nutritious and satisfying diet must

---

*Please check with your doctor before beginning a fast. Those with blood sugar problems may feel weak and dizzy as a result of a twenty-four-hour fast. These individuals are advised to begin by skipping one meal, or fasting just half a day. Once this shorter fast feels comfortable, they can safely undertake a twenty-four-hour fast.

be able to utilize the food we put in our mouths. The most perfect combination of foods will turn to fat if the body is not able to burn it off.

Food, we must remember, is body fuel. It is true that we derive great pleasure from eating. Yet beyond mere pleasure, food provides sustenance the body needs to perform. By merely feeding and fueling the body without demanding its exertion, we contribute to its idleness and hasten its deterioration. To have an optimal food experience we must give our bodies the exercise they need and deserve.

Think of your body as if it were a beloved pet. Every day take it out for a long walk. Throw a few sticks and let your body chase them. When you come home to dinner you will have a greater appreciation for both food and hunger.

TIPS ON SUPERIOR NUTRITION

Here are some specific techniques of how and what to eat.* These techniques are based on the simplest and most fundamental of natural laws. By studying them carefully you will begin to see how your present diet can be modified, how you can find the diet that will best meet your particular needs.

Once again the reader is asked not to be deceived by the simplicity of these ideas. They represent the careful refinement of hundreds of different nutritional concepts. They are the simplest, yet most effective, ways to find harmony with food.

*And please don't forget that any dietary changes should be made very slowly. You don't have to throw out your present diet. Keep it, and try to improve it. Many people are lured by diets that help them lose or gain weight in a hurry. Such extreme weight fluctuations can be harmful; they create ten-

---

*In-depth discussion of common nutritional questions is found in Appendix C, "Short Essays on Nutrition," page 163.

sion and stress. It may take several years to find a diet that is truly right for you. Meanwhile, you will be eating better and giving your body and mind a chance to enjoy the changes.

• *Certain fermented foods are a very important nutritional source.* These are fermented milk products, sauerkraut, and miso.

Fermented milk products such as buttermilk, yogurt, and kefir are extremely beneficial in aiding digestion. They help establish and maintain the important and protective intestinal flora that line the stomach.

Sauerkraut, made from cabbage, is an excellent and nutritious winter food.

Miso, or fermented soybean paste, is a high-protein seasoning and food. It can be used as a base for soups and other dishes.

• *Some foods have the effect of raising the body's general resistance.* They are especially important in winter, when there are more extreme changes in weather and people generally get less exposure to sunlight.

✳These important nutritional plants are garlic, parsley, watercress and garden cress, horseradish root, lemon, carrot, beet, cabbage, onion, sunflower sprouts, and buckwheat sprouts.

For optimal nutritional value, these plants should be eaten raw with as much of their edible components as possible. Horseradish root is very strong and should be blended with grated beets. Raw beets must be grated and slightly oiled, otherwise they can burn the throat. Raw garlic should be mashed and marinated for several hours in olive oil; it is easier to digest and does not damage the stomach.

• *Avoid eating rich foods.* They are hard to digest and tend to make us less sensitive to simple, more nutritious food.

Rich sauces, pastries, animal fats, and butter should be eaten in moderation. Two or three eggs per week is plenty.

Eat lean meats, poultry, and fish. Cut down on consumption of beef, pork, and lamb. Trim fat from meats before cooking. Avoid fried foods.

A baked potato is a nutritionally good food. It is relatively low in calories. When eaten as part of a good meal, with yogurt and chives or "buttered" with a little vegetable oil, it is an important food source. Yet this same baked potato eaten with gravy and butter is a less nutritious food, full of calories and saturated fats.

· *Sweeteners of all kinds should be used in moderation.*

Refined sugar is particularly hard on the body. Raw honey is preferable, though it too should be used moderately.

The natural sugar found in ripe fruit is the best sweetener. Dried fruits are laden with glucose but may be eaten in small quantities after you have reconstituted them by soaking them for several hours in fresh water.

· *Stimulants such as sugar, beer, tea, coffee, alcohol, tobacco, and drugs, including stimulating herbs such as ginseng, should be used in moderation.*

· *Use salt in moderation.*

Salt is found naturally in most foods. It is seldom necessary to add more. If you want additional salt, try sea salt or lake salt or, better yet, salty vegetables from the sea, such as dulse or kelp. These are readily available as powdered seasonings.

· *Eat a good, big breakfast.*

By eating a large, wholesome breakfast you will get the energy you need for the day and will be less tempted to snack and eat between meals. Begin the day by drinking two glasses of fresh water. Then eat some fresh fruit that is in season.

· *Children should be given salad as the first course, when their appetite is strongest and they are truly hungry.* The addition of a few currants or raisins, and/or small chunks of raw cheese, will help make the salad appetizing and enticing to an empty stomach. In this way children will learn to enjoy and appreciate fresh vegetables and develop good nutritional habits at an early age. (See Prime Rice au Raisin, page 79.)

• *Whatever you eat and drink — hamburgers or brown rice, french fries or baked potatoes, wine or carrot juice — must ultimately be satisfying to you.* Much of this satisfaction can come from getting personally involved with the food process: growing the food, preparing it, or even making some of the utensils. This preparation, whether it is growing a few sprouts in the kitchen or making your own jams and jellies, will greatly increase food satisfaction and contribute to a harmonious food rhythm.

RECIPES FOR A SMALL, HAPPY STOMACH

The recipes that follow are simple, yet complete and satisfying. They are designed to introduce you to foods that are tasty, nutritious, simple to prepare, and inexpensive. Each recipe has been chosen because it demonstrates one or more of the principles of superior nutrition discussed in this chapter. By reviewing this chapter carefully and learning to prepare some of the recipes, you will be better prepared to find your own version of nutritional harmony.

Many people who would thoroughly enjoy these foods in a restaurant are reluctant to eat them in their own homes. They are hesitant because the ingredients and directions are unfamiliar. Don't let this happen to you. Don't be discouraged because little cooking or baking is involved and because many familiar household foods, such as eggs, butter, salt, and sugar, are not included. You may be surprised and delighted to discover that there are many tasty ways to eat common fruits and vegetables. A simple carrot, for example, when grated and mixed with olive oil, lemon juice, and a few raisins, becomes a rich treat that can satisfy the most discriminating eater.

These recipes have been foraged from many different sources — grandmothers, mothers, fathers, friends, grandfathers, favorite uncles and aunts, and especially experience. Aside from being an enjoyable experience and tasting good (reason enough for their inclusion in this brief anthology of food), these dishes may also test and stretch your creativity, introducing you to new tastes, new foods, and new ways of combining well-known ingredients. Discover for yourself the exotic, exquisite taste of simple foods that are properly and harmoniously combined.

Try this simple recipe: Grate one large or two small apples in their entirety — with peel, core, some of the seeds, and the pulp. To this grated apple immediately add the freshly squeezed juice of one-eighth lemon or one teaspoon apple cider vinegar. Add a tablespoon of raw flaked oats that have been soaked for several minutes in fresh water, and a tablespoon of crushed, freshly shelled nuts. Mix the entire concoction carefully — the apple, oats, nuts, and lemon juice.

Close your eyes and sit up straight. Bring a spoonful of this simple fuel to your mouth. Slowly savor the incredible flavor of one of the most nutritious of all foods, pure, unfired, and simple — fit for the palate and vibrant health of both peasant and king.

Albert (alligator) to a rap at the door:

"Who's that knockin'
when I is practisin'
Makin' blueberry pies
outen carrots an oatmeal?"

—Pogo (*American comic strip*)

Breakfast

Blueberry Meusli

Take a handful of raw rolled oats (or roll your own by purchasing whole oat groats and flaking them in a blender) and cover with water for thirty minutes. They can be soaking while you get dressed and ready for the day. Add one-quarter cup sunflower seeds and freshly squeezed juice of one-eighth lemon (apple vinegar may be substituted for the lemon). To this add a generous portion of blueberries, or whatever fruit is available. Mix gently and enjoy.

Morning Tea

First warm the teapot by rinsing with hot water. Then add three teaspoons dried or fresh peppermint leaf. Pour boiling water over the leaves. Keep covered (grandmother used a tea cosy) and allow to steep for five to ten minutes.

While the tea is steeping, busy yourself in this manner: take two slices of your favorite whole wheat toast or cracker and spread generously with rosehip jam.

The tea, strained, is delightful with or without a spoonful of honey.

Lunch

There was an old doctor of some renown
Who coughed and sputtered like a basset hound
He examined himself and diagnosed croup
And wrote a prescription for garlic soup

–Lithuanian folk tale

Garlic Soup

Two cucumbers	Five cloves garlic
One pint yogurt	(six cloves for severe attack)
	Dash of sea salt

Dice cucumbers into fairly small pieces. Dilute yogurt in one pint cool water. Mix until there are no lumps. Add cucumber, garlic (which has been squeezed through a garlic press or finely chopped), and sea salt. Allow to stand for one hour.

Needless to say, the good doctor got better.

Midday Salad

Four persons are wanted to make a good salad — a philanthropist for oil, a miser for vinegar, a counselor for salt, and a madman to stir it all up.

—Ancient Chinese saying

Soak several handfuls of cracked wheat until soft (about one hour). Chop very fine: parsley, tomato, mint, cilantro (also called Chinese parsley and Mexican parsley), watercress, green onion, or any other fresh seasonal greens.

To this add the juice of several lemons, freshly squeezed; numerous cloves of garlic, squeezed through a garlic press or chopped very fine; and a liberal flow of best olive oil. Drain the water and add the wheat to the other ingredients. Add a dash of cayenne and mix until you find the perfect taste. Season with basil, oregano, thyme, etc.

If possible, allow to marinate for several hours before eating. Garlic should be used without discretion.

Note: Apple cider vinegar may be used instead of lemon juice, and a madwoman may be substituted for a madman.

Afternoon Snacks

Children of all ages love afternoon snacks (and morning and evening snacks too!). Next time you're feeling starved and want to break your between-meal fast, try one of the following.

Grapefruit for Four

Peel four grapefruits, the same way you would peel four oranges. Cut into bite-size chunks. Add sesame seeds and crushed walnuts, one-half cup each. Pour on one tablespoon maple syrup and two handfuls (one cup) finely chopped mint.

You may add ten finely chopped dates (without pits) instead of maple syrup — or with maple syrup if you have a sweet tooth to appease.

Walnut Delight

Chop two ounces each: figs, prunes, apricots, or any other delectable dried fruit. Soak until soft (at least one hour, preferably overnight) in water. Add two handfuls walnuts, the juice of one-quarter lemon, and a little raw honey.

The Evening Meal

The evening meal has traditionally been a time of celebration. The family is at last together — this is a perfect opportunity to share the day's experiences, relax, and enjoy some good wholesome food. To begin with, let us suggest a few appetizers. There is nothing like food to make one hungry!

Fingerlickin' Dip

Tofu is a delicious soft cheese made from soybeans. Besides being a superior source of protein, tofu is a superior taste treat. It may be purchased in many food stores or can be made in your own home (considerable work but worth the effort).

Mash one pound of tofu well. Add one-quarter cup best olive oil and the juice of one-quarter lemon, freshly squeezed, or two teaspoons apple cider vinegar. Add a child's handful of cumin seed, crushed, and a dash of soy sauce. Mix until all ingredients are evenly blended.

This is an exquisite dish. People who don't like tofu and think soybeans are for animals lap this up like puppies. This can be used as a dip, spread on toast, eaten with a spoon, used as a salad dressing, or enjoyed from the tip of a finger.

Chrain (to be made near an open window)

Horseradish root   Honey
Beet   Fresh air
Lemon juice

Take a deep breath. Grate four ounces (about as much as a medium-size carrot) fresh horseradish root and two ounces fresh beet. Add juice of one-half lemon and one tablespoon honey.

Serve with crackers, rye bread, or fresh carrot or celery sticks. Many people swear by it as the ideal condiment with meat or fish.

Instant Soup

Single serving: place one teaspoon miso in a small soupbowl. Fill bowl with boiling water. Stir until miso is thoroughly dissolved.

This broth is delicious and nutritious simply on its own. It's also a marvelous stock for adding favorite delicacies such as lightly sauteed mushrooms, leftover rice, chopped greens such as parsley, chives, and green onions, bread or cracker crumbs, and so on.

Note: Miso, which is made from soybeans, can be purchased in most natural food stores and in Japanese grocery stores.

Main Course: Prime Rice au Raisin

Grate equal portions of carrots and turnips. Add olive oil, fresh lemon juice, your favorite seasoning, raisins, and chunks of raw cheddar cheese. Now add brown rice which has been cooked with lentils (one-quarter cup lentils for each cup rice) and a bay leaf. Mix all ingredients with a wooden spoon, and serve in a wooden bowl.

Dessert: Jungle Salad
Into your favorite bowl put

Four ripe bananas, cut into rounds	Two handfuls seedless grapes or raisins (soaked)
Four crisp apples, cut in chunks	Juice of two oranges
	Juice of one-half lemon
Small pieces of soaked dried prunes	Dab of raw honey
	Nice portion of good yogurt

Top with crushed nuts. Makes enough for four children or two full-grown chimpanzees.

Nightcap

℞: to soothe tired minds and stomachs

One-quarter lemon: squeeze
the juice (or one teaspoon
apple cider vinegar)

One cup hot water
One-half teaspoon honey, to
taste

Stir, sip, relax, sleep.

To sleep easy all night
Let your supper be light
Or else you'll complain
Of a stomach in pain

—Mother Goose

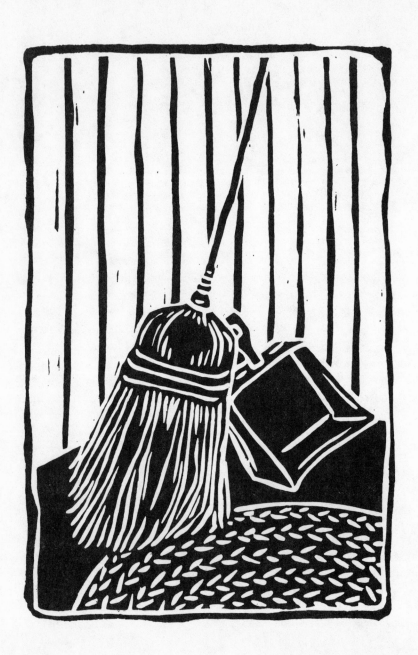

Chapter 6

℞: Good Housekeeping

THE HUMAN BODY is an engineering wonder. When functioning normally, its millions and millions of little parts all work together in harmony. And if something prevents one part from performing its duties, all the others rush to its aid and help out until it is whole and hearty again.

When we are cold, for example, we automatically shiver to produce heat. When we are hot, our pores open so we can sweat and cool down. When we are tired, our rhythm slows and we rest. When we are rested, we once again immerse ourselves in activity. When we are hungry, we seek food. When we are full and have the nourishment we need, our natural impulse is to empty ourselves through elimination.

Similarly, our mind continually seeks harmony among the divergent forces of the universe. We eagerly fill ourselves with dreams, notions, knowledge, ideas — with the wonders of life and creation. And when we have filled our emotional vessel, our instinct is to withdraw, to assimilate and digest this input of the larger world.

This balancing act, between activity and rest, hot and cold, emptiness and fullness, is always going on inside us. When we tip the scale too far in one direction, we are eventually forced to do something about it. This forced rebalancing generally takes the form of illness. When we are emotionally exhausted, we can no longer think straight; whether or not we like it, we must pull back from mental activity. On a physical plane, illness is often a forced withdrawal from activity — too much, not enough, or the wrong kind. At every moment, whether or not we are aware of it, the body and mind are responding in subtle ways to the flips and flops of daily living.

In the last chapter we discussed an important body fuel, solid food. We learned how to maximize our nutrition through selection, preparation, mastication, and so on. And just as we need and desire this solid food — to enrich the blood, to build muscle and bone — so too do we continually need to balance this input with regular output, or elimination.

Input, at least for most of us, poses no problem. We are constantly bombarded with information and choices — psychological fuel to run and even overrun our minds. Similarly, we have an abundance and often an overabundance of both appetite and food to satiate our desires and meet our body's needs for solid energy. Our problem is not how to get more input but how to temper its flow and eliminate it once it is ingested. Since elimination of excess involves a similar process be it food or ideas, let us now turn our attention to the elimination of solid food.

Most of us eat two, three, or even four meals a day, yet often have only one or two bowel movements. Moreover, we are often hungry and feel unsatisfied even after eating so many times. What happens to the food that is not eliminated? Could it in some way be responsible for the hollow, unsatisfied feelings we frequently get, the cravings long after bowls and bowls of food have been consumed?

Some of this food, of course, is absorbed into the body through the blood. But what is left, *excess fuel the body cannot use or store, becomes lodged within the vast appendages of the abdomen and stomach and encourages the spread of toxins from the bowel into the bloodstream. Many common and less common illnesses, including headaches, constipation, chronic diarrhea, cancer of the bowel, and depression (to name but a few), are associated with this incomplete elimination.

Several eliminative techniques, including sweating, drinking more water, and eating light, easily digestible food, are discussed in earlier chapters. In addition to these techniques, two other important things can be done to restore harmony between input and output of body fuel. The first is natural and proper toning and use of the abdominal muscles; the second is correct breathing and posture.

Of all the muscles of the body, the abdominals are surely the least used and most abused. This is due in part to our increasingly sedentary and machine-oriented way of living, which rarely calls for the use of abdominal muscles, and to the strain we place on these muscles through upright posture, improper diet, and overeating. This is unfortunate, because these muscles are vitally important to good health, affecting posture, digestion, and elimination as well as clothing size and vanity. Is it not true, for example, that after an especially large meal, when our bellies are full and distended, we tend to feel tired, sluggish, heavy, and possibly even irritable and a little depressed? And that following a good bowel movement we invariably feel lighter, more awake, more energetic, relaxed, vibrant, confident, open, creative — more alive?

Strong abdominal muscles carry the food we eat quickly and efficiently through the digestive tract. Weak abdominal muscles contribute to sluggish digestion and elimination: the food stays longer in the stomach, thus causing a persistent uneasy feeling in that area. Little wonder that the noun *relief* and verb *relieve* are associated with bodily function, or that it is through the stomach that we are first nourished and connected to our mothers, or that more than 90 percent of all illnesses and operations are specifically involved with this part of the human anatomy. It is surely not an overstatement to call the belly the center of the human anatomical universe.

Having established the significance of this neglected and important part of the body, let us see what we can do to keep it healthy, to "eliminate" any problems associated with it.

The first step in getting reacquainted is to learn and practice a simple exercise called the Abdominal Squeeze. This can be done sitting, standing, or lying down and can be practiced nearly anytime, anywhere — while driving down the freeway, sitting at a desk, standing in line at the grocery store, or lying in bed. Or even while reading this book! Why not try it right now? Here's how it works:

∗Inhale slowly through your nose, taking in as much air as possible. Then exhale through your mouth, squeezing as much air out of the lungs as possible. Try to do this slowly and rhythmically, without strain. This may take some practice, but eventually you should be able to place your hand on your abdomen and feel the air being squeezed out.

Once you have squeezed the air out, hold it out and draw up the abdominal wall (the region of the navel) energetically toward your chest. At the same time pull the abdomen as far back against your spine as possible. With practice you will form a cavity or hollow and your ribs will protrude.

Hold the pressure steadily for a few seconds, then relax your abdomen and inhale. Repeat five or six times, twice daily, gradually extending the cavity and holding it twenty or thirty seconds. Remember: pull in your abdomen as far as possible each time so that your internal organs get a good massage.

That's all there is to it! The Abdominal Squeeze, if practiced regularly and conscientiously, can have remarkable and far-reaching results. It will reacquaint you with your belly and help bring it back to life. This will take time, perhaps weeks or months, but eventually you will learn to control these muscles once again and your cavity will increase in size.

The effects? A stronger, firmer belly, less flab, easier elimination, improved circulation and better skin tone, better posture, general restoration and pulling up of all prolapsed organs, and most important, a keen sense of satisfaction at having gained control over a vital and important part of your body.*

The second technique to improve elimination is closely related to abdominal restoration; it is correct breathing and posture.

As upright, two-legged creatures we are at a considerable structural disadvantage. The legs, our base of support, simply do not provide us with much "grounding" or stability; as a result, we are very easily tipped over. Yet if we drop to hands and knees, on all fours, we have a much more solid base and are not easily upset and displaced. *This disruption of postural stability in many ways describes our emotions too. That is why a hobby like gardening, in which we bend over and place our hands in the earth, is often an effective therapy for emotional imbalance.

To improve our upright, two-legged posture, we must bring our bodies into muscular harmony and balance. The key to this improvement is full-body diaphragmatic or belly breathing plus a strong girdle of abdominal muscles that can support good upright posture.

First, about breathing. There are surely as many techniques as there are people, as many good theories as there are authors and experts, but the heart of the matter is this: most of the time we breathe too shallowly and too rapidly. By shallow I mean our in-breaths and out-breaths go only as far as the chest, whereas they should extend to the abdomen. This can be improved by becoming more aware of the breath, by listening to it and following its passage through the body. Practice breathing into different areas — for example, to the fingers, to the toes, to the knees. *With practice you will discover that you

* See also "Improving Elimination and Firming Abdominal Muscles," page 154.

can actually direct the breath where you like, and thereafter all breaths, whether at rest or during exertion, will pass in and out through the abdomen. We actually breathe through our bellies.

Also, practice breathing more slowly and rhythmically, gradually extending in-breaths and out-breaths to six or seven per minute. A good way to do this is to go for a walk and synchronize the breaths according to the steps you take. Or feel your pulse and monitor in-breath and out-breath according to your heartbeat. At first this increased attention to breath may feel somewhat awkward, but it is well worth the effort. Most of us have become shallow breathers without being aware of it. In time, longer, slower breaths will become second nature again, and there will no longer be need for practice and exercise of this normal body function.

Now, about posture. Posture, of course, is quite an individual matter. We are all constituted differently, with different weight distribution, bone mass, structure. We need different bodies according to the way we live, yet the need for good posture is universal — regardless of what we do or how we're built. And the secret to good posture is the same for all of us: an awareness of standing more upright, distributing our weight so we are not so easily upset and tipped over, pulling up our abdominal organs and chest while keeping our shoulders down. * Picture yourself standing tall, back straight, walking along carrying two heavy buckets of water. This will be good posture.

If we carry this postural awareness with us while sitting, driving, eating, and sleeping, we will gradually learn to assume it naturally. At first it will not be so easy. We are accustomed to slouching, and sagging abdominal muscles tire easily and are reluctant to support good upright posture. But persist. With practice you will get stronger, more confident, and comfortable with this new feeling.

Good posture, deep breathing, and strong abdominals have more benefits than just improved elimination and a better figure. ✳When we stand tall and our stomach feels strong and our breath is contented and controlled, we project a certain attitude and confidence about ourselves. When we feel tired and depressed, for example, we tend to sag and slouch and are more grumpy and irritable. When we feel confident and sure of ourselves, more open and receptive, we stand taller, our chest expands, and we are better able to deal with whatever the world sends our way.

The body we are born with, whether we like it or not, is our constant companion as we move through life. Through good times and bad times, happiness and unhappiness, slim and fat, youth and old age, it is always with us. It is like an eternal and irrevocable marriage vow: for better or worse, until death do us part. And no matter how estranged we may feel from our body, divorce is not possible. Even when we neglect it — when it huffs and puffs after but a few steps, when it sags under the burden of a rolypoly paunch, when it groans under the stress of marital upheaval and financial trauma — it is still the only body we will ever have, at least until we step out of it permanently.

Like a partner in any marriage, our body requires a certain amount of care and attention: it needs food, water, rest, activity, and an occasional pat here and there to assure it that it is loved and needed. Even those of us who have neglected our bodies can take comfort in the fact that the human organism is incredibly forgiving and has truly remarkable powers of rejuvenation. It seems to have a nearly boundless capacity to bounce back — from pain, injury, neglect — and is always ready to serve us on our journeys. Could one ever find a more devoted and faithful companion?

GOOD HOUSEKEEPING TIPS

1. Better to do a little cleaning each day than a lot of cleaning all at once. When dirt piles up it is much more difficult to remove. Don't expect an accumulation of many years to disappear overnight.

2. In some instances, when a house has not been cleaned for many years, the waste may be piled so high that it is not readily removed through the gentle cleansers suggested in this chapter. In this case it may be necessary to use tools with a little more clout, such as an enema or a colonic, which can rather dramatically remove years of debris. They should only be used as emergency or temporary expedients, though, as they are external measures and do not really teach you to clean your own home. Once they have helped with the major cleanup, get busy and use the daily house-cleaning techniques recommended in this book — drinking more water, eating properly, maintaining good posture, breathing deeply, sweating, and daily exercising the abdominal muscles.

3. *Major cleanup can also be facilitated by drinking hot water instead of customary room-temperature water. Drink two cups upon rising and one every hour throughout the day. When cleanup has been completed, which usually takes three or four days, begin drinking room-temperature water again.

4. Fasting one day a week is a wonderful way to clean house without doing much work. The house cleans itself! Of course this kind of weekly maintenance cleanup will only be really effective if the home is kept reasonably clean all the time. It's like giving the maid the day off.*

5. Even after you begin a regular daily program of house-cleaning, a seasonal cleanup or longer fast is highly rec-ommended. The seasonal fast generally lasts three or four

* For fasting precautions, see footnote, page 70.

days and only water is ingested, though you may add a few drops of vinegar or lemon juice to the water if desired. Those with no previous fasting experience should begin with shorter fasts, twenty-four to forty-eight hours, and if drinking only water proves too difficult, you can substitute vegetable or fruit juice diluted fifty-fifty with water.

6. Refuse that refuses to leave can often be coaxed out by use of a gentle plant, psyllium seed. This is available in many natural food stores and herbal apothecaries and should be used whenever possible in its whole form, preferably the blond whole seed. It is also readily available in commercial pharmacies as Metamusil, though this and similar brands are made from the powdered plant and are not as efficacious as the whole seed. For best results, take two teaspoons with water every three hours for two or three days. This gentle "broom" is highly effective in removing persistent debris, the kind you would not be likely to come upon during normal cleaning. Remember, though, it is not to be used regularly and does not replace the need for daily cleaning.

7. The art of relaxation, as discussed in Chapter 2, can greatly facilitate good elimination. So often our bellies get tight; we actually carry tension in the solar plexus. This frequently results from being in a hurry to move the bowels, not taking enough time to relax and perform this important bodily function properly. As schoolchildren we are often hesitant to ask permission to leave the class, encouraged by classmates and teachers to wait. This "holding," whether in school or later in home or office, is a very poor habit: the body soon learns to ignore the call of nature. The result: a gradual diminution of peristaltic action and fewer bowel movements. So, when going to the toilet, take your time, relax, breathe deeply. Give elimination your full attention and enjoy this important part of the eating ritual.

8. No matter how clean we keep our internal house, we will never enjoy really natural elimination if we continually overeat, especially late in the day. Too much fuel — even the very best quality — overloads the system and puts a heavy burden on the eliminative organs. ✻A simple way of correcting this problem is "meal reversal" — eat the large meal during the day and a very light meal in the evening. Or skip the evening meal altogether. This gives the body time to process and eliminate the food before you go to sleep. You will sleep better and wake up feeling more rested.

9. Another way to improve elimination is to use the squatting position rather than the normal sitting position while moving the bowels. This requires practice, strong legs, and good balance; most of us are not accustomed to using our bodies in this way, and modern toilets are not designed for this kind of use. Nevertheless, learning to squat in this manner is well worth the effort, as it can often help overcome persistent eliminative difficulties. Best results are generally obtained by squatting on the toilet bowl rather than the toilet seat, or by resting the feet on a strong wooden stand or platform approximately ten inches high while defecating from the usual seated position on the toilet seat.

    This squatting position is the most natural for elimination, as it ensures the bowel is open and the full benefit is derived from peristaltic action. Though little practiced in modern times, it is still used in many parts of the world and is a standard in most "primitive" cultures, where people cannot afford modern plumbing or laxatives — and do very well without either.

10. One final word: please do not become too fanatical about housecleaning. Some people are forever looking here and there for obscure pieces of dirt. They spend half their life dieting, fasting, taking purgatives and flushes, preaching the virtues of cleaning to anyone who will listen, and gen-

erally alienating themselves from the world with their
housecleaning obsession. Housecleaning is best done slowly,
quietly, regularly, without fanfare: simply let the body do
its own gentle work. There is no need to talk about it, even
with friends. The results will speak for themselves. When
you feel better inside you will look better outside. Your
skin, your posture, your good humor, and your happiness
will radiate how you feel.

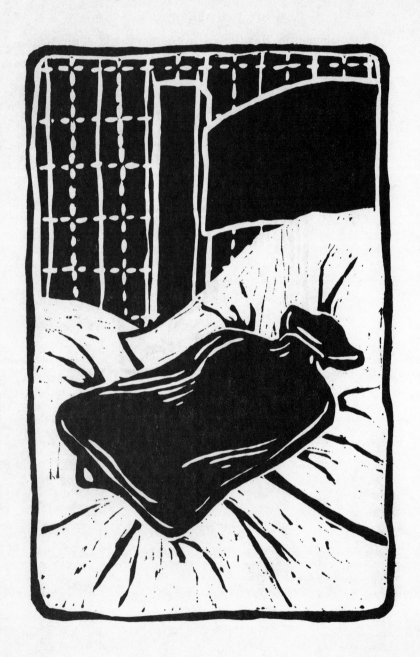

Chapter 7

Rx: Old-Fashioned Remedies for Modern-Day Ailments

SOMETIMES we get so involved with complicated solutions to everyday problems that we overlook simple, ordinary things that can help us feel better. These simple remedies are really just good old common sense. But since most of us tend to be slightly forgetful, a reminder is sometimes helpful.

> He best will live who will arrange
> His way of life to constant change
>
> —Mother Nature

These prescriptions may remind you of your grandparents or other "old-fashioned" people you may have met, heard about, or read about. This is good. These older people often have a quiet wisdom that penetrates beyond the sophistication of our modern-day lives. In their simplicity we may discover or rediscover something that can make our own lives easier and more enjoyable, every day.

Cold Feet and the Hot Water Bottle

This is an old saying: "When your feet get cold, put your hat on." This is good advice.

The head is the body's radiator: it is through the head that much of the body's heat escapes. This adage might also have said, "Put your scarf on," because it is through the unprotected neck that cold air and chilling winds often penetrate the body. Many colds and minor illnesses can be prevented by wearing a hat and a wool scarf.

The best way to protect the body from cold is to wear several layers of light clothes. This is more effective than one heavy garment; the air between the layers acts as insulation. This layering has another advantage: it enables you to peel off your clothes as your body temperature rises. These extra clothes can be put aside or tied around your waist if you are walking. It is also wise to use an all-cotton, all-wool, or silk garment as the first layer; these natural fibers allow the body to breathe.

Wearing warm sweaters and jerseys is also a good alternative to turning up the thermostat in your home. Not only will you be saving energy, you will be contributing to your good health. Rooms that are overheated tend to dry the skin and discourage the body from generating its own heat. *Cool air stimulates the body to produce heat and encourages the circulation of fresh blood. Besides, when your skin feels slightly cool you are more likely to move around, and this movement is good for the circulation.

In general, when the body thermostat is working normally, the head is slightly cool and the feet are slightly warm. This is a normal, healthy balance. When you don't feel well — during a headache or fever, for example — you may notice that this is reversed: the head is warm and the feet are cool. *To return the body to its normal, healthy temperature polarity, you must

cool the head and warm the feet. Many people do this intu-
itively, putting a cool washcloth on their forehead and soaking
their feet in warm water. This is the proper way to help the
body return to its normal equilibrium: heat the feet and cool
the head.

This leads us to the hot water bottle, a useful and simple
home remedy which was more popular in Grandmother's time.
Not only does a hot water bottle warm cold feet, but it also
soothes stiff, sore necks, aching backs, and grumbling tum-
mies. The hot water bottle should be revived — taken out of
drawers and closets and restored to its place of honor in the
household.

Foot Comfort

There was a sign outside a large warehouse. It said: "If you
want to worry more, wear tight shoes." This is very good
advice.

How many times have you heard the expression "My feet
are killing me"? Who doesn't enjoy coming home, taking off
the shoes, and going barefoot or wearing soft slippers? The
way we abuse our feet is really a crime. Tight shoes and high
shoes are stylish but they hurt. And they contribute to tension
and irritability. That goes for tight anything — pants, under-
garments, belts. There is nothing stylish about being uncom-
fortable.

Our feet are very important in our lives. Leonardo da Vinci
called the foot the greatest engineering device in the world.
Our feet do an incredible amount of work for us. Why do we
not give them the same love and concern we do the rest of our
body? When we were children our feet were healthy and happy.
Look at a baby's foot. You will see how mobile the toes are:
constantly gripping, stretching, and bending. In fact, they are

remarkably like the hands, with nearly the same spread and range of movement.

The way to recapture the healthy feet of your childhood is to give them more love and attention. Let them go barefoot more often, even if it is only in your own home, on the carpet. Also, expose them to the air by wearing sandals occasionally so your toes can "breathe."

Give your feet some exercise and stimulation by wiggling them more. ✳ Each time you are ready to put on your socks, pick them up with your toes. Once this pleasant habit is established you will enjoy good toe exercise every day.

Buy shoes that are extra long and extra wide. At first they will feel big and sloppy, but this feeling will soon be replaced with comfort and satisfaction, because this sloppiness lets your feet breathe and allows your toes to wiggle and squirm.

The combination of concrete and tight shoes has ruined many peoples' feet and health. Cement does not give beneath the feet; therefore, it is important to wear shoes that give the maximum possible protection from hard surfaces. Purchase shoes that cushion the impact.

Acknowledging that your feet are important is a good first step in improving your foot comfort and health. Feet must be treated with respect. You will be pleasantly surprised to discover that your feet are really good friends. When they are happy, you will be happy.

Traveling

In the good old days people used to get very tired from traveling. Sometimes their feet would be sore from walking, or their bottoms would be bruised from bouncing up and down on the seat of a horse-drawn wagon. Or they might be stiff and aching from jostling in the saddle for many hours.

Even though travel today is much more comfortable and convenient, it can still be a very exhausting experience, and often leaves us stiff and grumpy. Being in one position for several hours means we do not get the stimulation needed for good circulation. As a result, our blood pools in certain areas, thus contributing to our discomfort. This pooling can and should be alleviated.

If you are taking a long car journey, make frequent stops to walk, stretch, stamp the feet, and get the blood circulating again. If children are traveling with you, a jump rope is a welcome friend for rest stops. These stretch breaks will not only keep you from getting stiff and tired but will make your journey easier and safer.

Car journeys frequently cause back and shoulder pain because of the continuous pressure from sitting in the driving position. This is compounded because most automobiles do not have seats that adequately support the spine. ✳This discomfort can be avoided by placing a pillow, folded towel, or blanket in the small of the back and by making a special effort not to lean on the seat in such a way that the spine bends. It is this bending that causes the discomfort and can eventually lead to serious back problems.

Those who ride long distances in cars should also wiggle and move as much as possible, let in plenty of fresh air, and encourage other passengers to massage the head, neck, and shoulders of the driver, who is the least mobile. Similarly, bus passengers should go for walks whenever the bus stops for a while.

Airline passengers, of course, are not able to get out every hour and go for a walk. They can, however, walk frequently in the aisles and even stretch a few times without attracting undue attention. Airline travelers are also vulnerable to the "time-stress factor," from moving rapidly through time and space. These rapid and dramatic changes — beginning a journey in a hot climate and arriving a few hours later in a cold climate, for example — require careful adjustment. *The best thing you can do after a long air journey is to go for a long walk. Then take a short nap. This gives the body and mind the time they need to acclimate to changes of weather, time, people, etc.

Tooth Care

There are many theories about how best to care for the teeth. What follows is a simple, effective way to prevent tooth decay and gum deterioration.

*Get in the habit of rinsing your teeth with water after every meal or snack. Swish the water round and round in your mouth, swirling it against the gums, gargling, then spitting. Repeat this two or three times. This will effectively rid the teeth of potentially harmful bacteria and, if practiced carefully, help prevent cavities.

Use dental floss at least once a day. Clean between the teeth, getting out all the lodged particles the water can't reach. Be sure to use the floss gently; it is possible to injure the gums by forcing the floss into the crevices between teeth.

Using a modest amount of toothpaste or toothpowder, gently brush the teeth. Brush vertically, placing the bristles on the gums above the teeth and brushing down. Remember, this motion should be gentle and can be done by holding the toothbrush like a pencil. Be sure the toothbrush is fairly soft so the bristles will not scrape and injure the gums. The purpose of this brushing is a very mild stimulation of the gums as well as a cleaning of the teeth.

The importance of proper exercise and stimulation of the teeth must not be overlooked. Just like any other part of the body, the teeth need exercise. Much of this exercise, of course, comes from eating: by chewing the food, the gums and teeth are stimulated, which brings fresh blood to all areas of the mouth. This kind of exercise appears easy: everyone loves to eat. But the problem is that much of the popular processed food does not require the kind of mastication that brings fresh blood to the teeth and gums. Furthermore, eating fast and swallowing the food before it has been thoroughly masticated deprives the teeth of important stimulation and exercise.

Proper stimulation comes from chewing fresh, raw fruits and vegetables such as carrots and apples. The old saying "An apple a day keeps the dentist at bay" is more than just a fable. Apples clean the teeth and at the same time provide the kind of exercise the teeth need to be healthy and cavity-free.

Sleeping

Sleeping is one of the most enjoyable and important human activities. We spend over one-third of our lives in bed, and how we feel when we get out of bed can determine how we feel the rest of the day. Do you wake up feeling rested? Do you sometimes feel tired even after sleeping eight or nine hours? Do you sometimes wake up with a stiff neck or a sore back? If so, you might want to consider some important and often overlooked facts about sleeping.

For one thing, you should be aware that the hours you actually sleep are very important. That is, the eight hours between 10:00 P.M. and 6:00 A.M. have a different rest potential than the eight hours between 2:00 A.M. and 10:00 A.M. In each case the total sleeping time is eight hours, but the quality of the rest can be markedly different. In general, the closer your sleep rhythm approximates the day/night rhythm, the more restful your sleep will be. Going to bed at 11:00 P.M. and rising

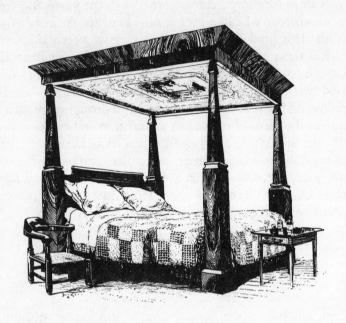

at 7:00 A.M. will leave you more rested and refreshed than going to bed at 1:00 A.M. and getting up at 9:00 A.M.

Of course this varies with individuals and with seasons. It is possible to become a more nocturnal person by using electric lights to alter day/night rhythm. It is also true that many of our daily activities are not designed to reflect the changes of day and night brought by the different seasons.

There are other important factors that influence the quality of sleep. The surface we sleep on may be too soft, not giving our body the support it needs to rest adequately. Sleep on a firm surface; put a board under the mattress if necessary.

✳The position in which we sleep can also greatly influence our sleep. Sleeping on the side with one knee drawn up, as illustrated in the prescription that follows, is perhaps the best sleeping posture.

A good way to improve your sleep is to have the window slightly open. Turn down the heat in your room and put on extra blankets so you will not be cold. This fresh air is very important. For eight hours you will be taking in good, fresh oxygen, and this promotes total, restful sleep.

The subject of sleep is very personal, of course. Six hours may be adequate for one person and not enough for another. Then too, modern "night life" works against going to bed early: many interesting and important activities take place long after the chickens have gone to bed. Still, despite these pleasant disturbances, it is possible to modify our schedules so that we benefit more from the third of our lives we spend in bed.

The best way to find out what works for you is to do a little experimenting. Try sleeping on a little bit harder surface. Try going to bed an hour earlier and getting up an hour earlier. Try putting on an extra blanket and opening the window an inch or two. You may be pleasantly surprised to find yourself waking up more rested and relaxed, better prepared for the day.

THE ART OF A GOOD NIGHT'S SLEEP

The sleep/relaxation technique described below will help you sleep better and wake up more fully rested. If done properly it will strengthen the spine and improve your posture.

At first it may feel awkward. Persevere. After a few nights or naps you will get used to the new position and wake up with the satisfied feeling of a complete and restful repose.

1. Lie on your back. Draw up your right knee and at the same time raise your arms to shoulder level.

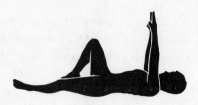

2. Roll over bodily to the left side with your arms descending. The left leg lies relaxed and the right crosses it comfortably; your arms lie limply across your body. A pillow placed between the bent top knee and the bed makes this easier, especially for those with lower back problems.

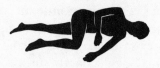

3. Now place a small pillow or cushion under your head only, taking care *not* to place it under your neck or shoulder. The pillow may be doubled to ensure better alignment of head and spine. If the pillow is placed properly, your head should be tilted slightly backward and your chin lifted slightly as though you were looking straight ahead.

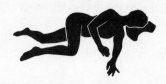

4. At this moment your head is in a continuous line with your spine, the perfect position for all daily activities. Take care not to lie on your upper arm; you should be resting firmly on the bony shoulder blade, broad and flat to take your weight.

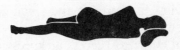

5. If you prefer to lie on the right side or change positions as you sleep, this position can be switched, merely reversing directions.

Sweet dreams . . .

Back Care

If you are like most people, you have trouble with your back from time to time. Back problems are notoriously painful and difficult to resolve. It is not uncommon for a person to suffer excruciating back pain and find out that nothing is medically wrong. Such is the nature of the spine.

Many back problems and back injuries can be avoided by learning a few simple techniques about proper care of the spine. These techniques help keep the spine flexible and healthy. It has often been observed that people are as healthy as their spines are flexible. So to stay healthy and enjoy a supple, responsive spine, consider the following tips.

Learn and follow a daily stretching routine such as that on page 146. This will help keep you supple and prevent most back injuries.

Try to avoid standing or sitting in one position for a long period of time. If you can't avoid it, do some wiggling and moving so that you do not get too stiff. *If you must stand in one place for a long time, elevate one foot by placing it on any raised object — the rung of a chair, a wastebasket, or anything else that is handy. Bar stools are especially made with this in mind; they make it possible for patrons to elevate one foot, thus relieving pressure on the spine and encouraging people to spend more time near the bar.

Make a special effort to keep your knees slightly bent and relaxed. Whenever you think of it, flex your knees slightly. This relieves pressure on your back and helps keep the spine in good upright posture.

When you sit in a chair, sit away from the back so that you are not leaning. Sit up straight with your legs squarely on the floor in front of you or crossed at the ankles. *Avoid sitting with one leg crossed on top of the other as this puts a strain on the spine and cuts off circulation by putting pressure on the blood vessels.

At first you may find these new positions difficult because the muscles needed to support the spine may be weak from inactivity. Be persistent. After a few weeks you will find that you can sit up without leaning. For this you will be rewarded with a stronger, more responsive spine.

Whenever you walk, lift your knees high. There is a strong tendency to shuffle the feet when walking, so the feet never really leave the ground or leave it ever so slightly. By lifting your legs from the thigh as you walk, you will automatically straighten the spine and improve your posture.

Try it. Stand up. Concentrate on the muscles in the front of your thigh from your pelvis to your knee. These are the ones that do the lifting. Lift up one leg from the thigh. Move it upward and forward and then put it down. Then lift up the other leg from the thigh and put it down. This is good walking. Walk two or three times around the room, lifting each foot from the thigh, keeping your toes pointed straight ahead so the feet do not splay in or out. You will feel the difference: your spine is straighter; your posture is better. With practice you will feel more graceful and relaxed. Your back will appreciate the difference.

At one time or another you have probably been told to bend your knees before lifting, but by now you may have forgotten. Remembering this one simple rule — even if it is merely bending to pick up a pencil — can prevent many serious back injuries. Always, always lift with your knees.

And once the object is in your hands, whether it is an orange or an elephant, keep your back straight and walk the same way you do when not loaded down. This spares your back and also allows you to carry a heavier load a longer distance before you tire.

When two people are lifting something, it is important that both people bend their knees and lift at the same time. Injuries frequently occur in such situations because one person lifts too fast, thus putting more of the weight and strain on the other person. Even though this person's knees are properly bent, he or she may be injured by the excess strain and load.

When carrying something on your shoulder or in your arms, don't always use the same side of your body. This goes for babies, handbags, groceries, and bottles of wine. If you do, you will eventually suffer back problems because of the uneven strain you are putting on your back and shoulder muscles.

Another useful way to prevent back injury and strain is to use a hanging bar, commonly called a chin-up bar. By simply hanging for a few seconds each day — with arms fully extended — your spine will elongate and relax, gradually recovering from the compression caused by sitting in chairs and automobiles. These adjustable hanging bars, made to fit any doorway, may be purchased in many sporting goods stores, or you can make your own, or hang from the limb of a friendly tree, the way children do.

Finally, a good way to prevent back strain, or to alleviate it, is to take a daily walk — on all fours. Do this "crabwalk" with your knees off the ground, using only your hands and feet to propel your body. Walking in this manner, like our animal friends, gives welcome relief to a tired spine and helps strengthen important muscles needed for normal upright posture.

Remember, too, that the cause of most back injuries is tension, the inability to relax. To avoid back problems, it is important to take time to relax. Slow down. Catch your breath. Close your eyes for a few seconds. Like any good horse, you should be turned out to pasture for at least a few minutes each day!

Try to avoid situations that contribute to your tension and fatigue. ✳Shrug your shoulders a few times during the day so no problems can perch on them. Rotate your head from side to side so no evil thoughts can lodge between your ears. Try at all times to keep yourself as loose, limber, and relaxed as you can. Learn to be lazy occasionally.

Saline Rinse and Gargle

At one time salt was considered the most valuable of all commodities: it was carried by camel across the great deserts and traded for precious stones and great piles of gold. Today, of course, salt has been relegated to a much less glamorous position. Though used liberally in most food preparations, it is considered somewhat harmful, and we are often well advised to use it much more moderately.

There is, however, a centuries-old method of using sea salt to clean the mouth, throat, and nasal passages. ✳This simple technique, the Saline Rinse and Gargle, is well worth learning and practicing, for it can strengthen gums and prevent sinus problems, and is a wonderful preventative for colds and sore throats. Here's how it works:

First, add a pinch of sea salt to a half glass of tepid water, taking care that the water is only about as salty as tears; otherwise it will irritate. Gargle thoroughly three or four times, swilling the water back and forth in your mouth so your teeth and gums are thoroughly irrigated. While gargling, hold the water in the back of your throat as long as possible. This is relatively easy: I have seen children as young as two years old do it with ease and enthusiasm. For best results, gargle in the evening, just before bed, or several times daily when you feel the onset of a cold or sore throat.

Now put a little saltwater in the palm of your left hand, close your right nostril by pinching it shut with your right thumb, and gently sniff the saltwater solution into your left nostril. At first you should allow the water to bubble at the nostril: in this way only a small quantity will be drawn in, and you will get accustomed to the practice. As you get used to it, roll your head back and draw in more water so that it passes through your nose and into your throat. When this is done, you may then eject the water through your mouth.

Do the same thing on the other side; put some saltwater in the palm of your right hand, close off your left nostril with your left thumb, and inhale through your right nostril.

This ancient form of nasal hygiene is simple, safe, and highly effective. Those who practice it regularly will be well repaid for their efforts. A few grains of sea salt can be worth ounces of gold in promoting better everyday health.

Eyestrain

It is rare for a person to go through life without eyestrain and spectacles, yet this is understandable when we consider the tremendous demands we place on our eyes — to read, to help us weave through busy traffic, to watch television.

Although not all eyestrain can be avoided, there are some things you can do to prevent the frequency of such strain. There are also a few things you can do when your eyes feel overtired.

To prevent eyestrain, it is a good idea to give your eyes periodic rests, short reprieves from all the focusing and concentration. The best way to do this is to close your eyes more often, even if it is only for a few seconds at a time. This can be done by simply closing your eyes, taking short naps, or, if you have a minute or so, palming.

*Palming is a simple, effective way of giving your eyes a nap. It works like this. Remove glasses or contact lenses. Rub the palms of your hands together until they are good and warm, almost burning, then quickly cup them and place them over your closed eyes, taking care not to press the eyes themselves. Hold the cupped palms over your eyes for one minute, allowing the warmth and darkness to penetrate and soothe the eyes. Afterward your eyes will feel greatly relaxed, grateful for this small attention.

Nearly everyone has had the experience of pinching the upper bridge of the nose, in the space between the eyes. This is a familiar and well-known way of reducing eyestrain: it relieves tension in the head. Try it. Right now, as you are reading this, remove your glasses or contact lenses. Apply pressure in the area by squeezing with the thumb and forefinger. You may notice that it becomes harder to concentrate on the words. In fact, reading becomes less interesting. This is fine. Take the opportunity to not-read for a few minutes.

One further hint on relief from eyestrain. Next time your eyes feel tired or strained, try alternately blinking and squeezing. Blink very rapidly three or four times, then close your eyes tight. Then blink three or four more times and squeeze again. Repeat this alternate blinking and squeezing a half-dozen times.

Finish by leaving the eyes closed and relaxed for one minute. Many people find great relief from eyestrain by using this simple technique.

And don't forget about our old friend cool water. Simply splashing cool water in the eyes when they feel tired or strained can often give almost instant relief.

Whatever techniques we use to rest our eyes, we should remember how important our eyes are. Sometimes we regard our vision so casually, forgetting how beautiful and unique it is. The ability to see and perceive things with the eyes is a very special gift. We should give our eyes the care they need and deserve. If we close them more often, they will be even more responsive when they are open.

Green Energy

Indoor plants are good for the health. They give off pleasing odors and are enjoyable to observe and nurture. They also keep the air fresh by absorbing carbon dioxide and giving off oxygen. Homes that are filled with green plants have fresher air, and the occupants of such houses benefit by feeling more alive and invigorated.

It is not expensive to fill your home with this kind of green energy. These plants need not be exotic; many of the native plants that grow in your area can be dug up and transplanted into containers for your home.

You can also grow a beautiful indoor garden by raising sunflower sprouts.* This is done in the following manner: * Obtain a small wooden flat, about three or four inches high, the kind fruits and vegetables come in. Line it with newspaper, then fill

* Note: You can sprout buckwheat in a similar manner using "sprouting buckwheat," seed with the hull still intact.

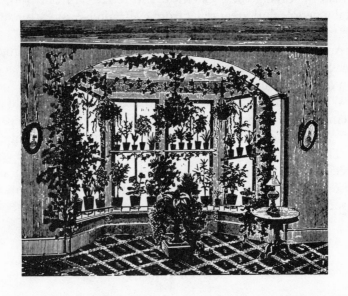

it with soil from which you have removed all large twigs and rocks. Smooth the soil out along the top of the box by "plowing" it gently with your fingers. Then moisten the soil by sprinkling it thoroughly with water.

Purchase some plain, unsalted, uncooked sunflower seeds which still have their outer hulls or shells intact. Soak them in water for twenty-four hours.

After the seeds are soaked, take them out of the water and broadcast them over your recently plowed and watered field of dirt. They can be as close as you like, even touching if they happen to fall that way.

Now take a piece of cloth and soak it in cool water. Place this cloth over the seeds so that the entire field is covered. For the next few days keep the cloth wet by pouring water over it a few times a day. One day you will notice that the cloth is being pushed up. This means the sunflowers have sprouted. Your garden is growing!

Remove the covering and say hello to your sprouts. Move them near some sunlight. Water them gently every day. Watch them grow. You will be amazed at how fast they push up, sometimes growing a half-inch or more before your eyes. Share this experience with children and other friends.

When the sprouts are five or six inches tall they are ready to eat. You can harvest them by pulling them up by their stems or by cutting them down near ground level with a knife, your sunflower scythe. They are nutritious and delicious, an exotic addition to a salad or just a quick munch. Children love them as "Sunflower Snacks."

Growing sunflower greens is a wonderful education. It affords you the opportunity to garden in your own home. It gives you nourishing food that has been grown with your own hands. It freshens and improves the air you breathe.

Charles Darwin, a great naturalist, studied the sunflower for many years. He observed that during the day the flowers of this beautiful plant slowly turned their heads, following the passage of the sun across the sky. This movement, called heliotropism, has come to mean the bending and turning of plants and people toward the sun's light.

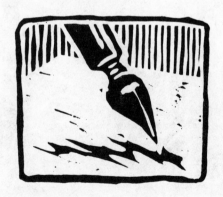

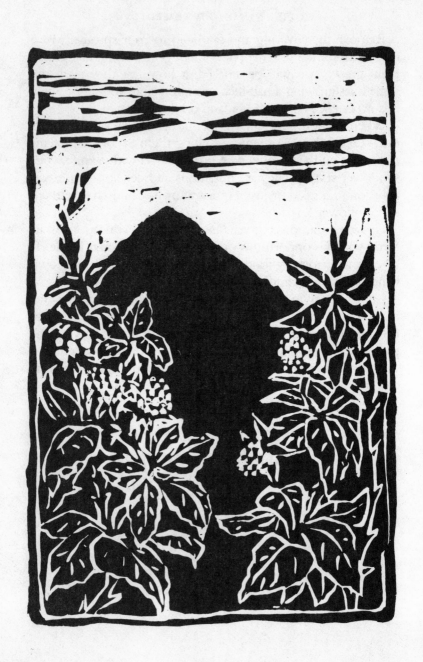

Chapter 8

℞: The Mountain of Youth

A YOUNG MAN in very poor health consulted all the most famous and learned doctors in the country. After giving him many complicated and sophisticated tests, the doctors told him that he had an extremely rare disease and would live only a few more weeks. They advised him that his only possible hope was to consult an old man who had been known to cure people suffering from the most incurable diseases. This old man, they said, lived on top of the highest mountain in the most rugged, inaccessible part of the country.

The young man was extremely frail from the long illness. His legs were spindly, his torso brittle and gaunt, yet he had a strong will to live. With the help of family and friends he assembled a small pack of provisions. Transportation was arranged to the base of the mountain, just where a narrow, blackberry-lined trail began. It was midsummer. The sun was hot. The youth picked a few berries, put them in his mouth, and, with feelings of both fatigue and resolution, started up the mountain.

The first few days were difficult and discouraging for the young man. His mind was determined, but his body resisted. Breaths were difficult: he never seemed to get sufficient air in his lungs to last until the next breath. His feet ached from the unaccustomed work; they became tender and swollen from the sharp stones that pushed against his thin shoes. But he persisted, climbing a few more feet each day, sucking blackberries and soaking his aching feet in cool mountain water from the stream that flowed alongside the trail. Whenever he stopped to soothe his tired feet, he also splashed cool water in his eyes and across his face. Gradually the splashing of cool water became one of his greatest pleasures; afterward he always felt invigorated and his enthusiasm for the journey was renewed. In this manner he proceeded, slowly gathering strength until, after a few weeks, he could actually cover a full mile during the day.

By this time his food supply had dwindled to almost nothing, for it had never occurred to him, or his family, that the journey would be so long and difficult. During the first weeks, while he was still close to civilization, he occasionally met goat herders who gave him a little cheese and bread. But this was infrequent and later he saw no one. Out of necessity he began to gather wild foods: greens, nuts, berries, and fruits. At first he felt half starved by this severely limited diet, but as he became stronger he learned to make the food more nourishing by chewing it longer. He also drank large quantities of fresh mountain water, which helped satisfy his hunger and gave him nourishment.

Gradually, almost imperceptibly, the days lengthened into weeks and months. Fortunately, the young man had brought along an extra layer of clothes, for now the days were shorter and cooler and he had to keep moving to stay warm. As winter approached he slept in caves or hollowed-out tree stumps, and he became very skilled at finding warm, dry shelter for the night. Because the nights were cold and often stormy, he went to bed early and was on the trail again with the very first sunlight.

The trail, which before had been easy to follow, had now

become overgrown with wild plants and slippery with mud. Under these difficult conditions the young man was forced to rely more and more on his instincts. He became a keen observer of plants and animals that shared this isolated hermitage; he learned to know when storms were coming by the smell of the air; he learned to recognize the habits of various insects and animals by observing disturbances and minute changes in the vegetation; he learned to walk quietly, almost soundlessly, so as not to frighten these creatures with his presence; he learned, too, that if he rubbed his skin and clothing with certain wild plants, his body odor became more like that of the mountain.

The winter passed slowly, and out of it grew the spring. The young man had never spent so much time alone; his only companions were the animals whose trails he followed and a friendly bird that seemed to be following him up the mountain. His mind occasionally wandered back to family and friends below, but the daily work of climbing the mountain and surviving kept him too occupied to live long in the past. In moments of doubt or frustration he thought of the old man on top of the mountain who might be able to cure him. This vision provided constant inspiration to continue the difficult journey.

The top of the mountain was flat like a tabletop and seemed to be a haven for hawks, which circled overhead, swiftly rising with the thermal drafts, then slowly drifting down, rising, then drifting again. They were as calm and light as the wind itself, and the young man spent a long time just lying on his back watching them perform this beautiful dance.

The clouds, too, were magnificent and fluffy, drifting by and through him until he began to feel as close to the heavens as he did distant from the earth. This was a time of silence and reflection.

The tabletop was not large. The young man tramped back

and forth across it, looking behind rocks and piles of brush, shouting as loud as he could so the old man he had come to see would know he had arrived. But there was no sign of life, only the echo of his own voice, which bounced off the rocks and came eerily back to his own ears. In fact, there was no sign of anyone living here before; he found no tracks, no shelter, nothing to indicate that the earth or vegetation had been disturbed by the presence of man.

At first the young man felt angry and keenly disappointed; he cursed the old man for not being there and stamped his feet angrily against the hard earth. He had gone to so much trouble to get here and now there was no one to consult, no one to cure him of his terrible illness. But after a few days of futile search and worry, he ceased to think so much about the old man and reflected instead on the calmness and serenity he now felt. It was so new, this feeling, something he had never experienced. Life below had been filled with so much suffering and stress, and the journey so long and difficult, that it was a great relief just to relax and enjoy the tranquility of the mountain. Besides, he was too busy to dwell long on his disappointment or loneliness. There was daily foraging to be done, and he found a hive of wild honeybees living in a tree stump; from them he took a little honey, leaving enough so the bees would still have plenty to eat in winter. He also dried currants and blackberries and built a small hut out of branches and sod.

In this manner he passed season after season. The past became the present, and soon he could remember it only through certain incidents on the mountain: the spring when he saw an airplane in the distance; the summer when a swarm of bees landed on the branch of a pine tree; the autumn when the deer began eating out of his hands; the winter that he built a snow house; that same winter, when several deer died of starvation. Life was not easy, but it was full; though it was not a life he

would have chosen, he accepted this situation and the fact that
it was his.

One day, many years later, the young man heard human voices
coming from the side of the mountain. He felt very excited
and ran here and there trying to see where the voices were
coming from, trying to imagine whom they might belong to.
He also felt afraid. So accustomed had he become to the sounds
of wind and the songs of birds that the noises that now came
to his ears seemed strange and frightening. It had been so long
since he had spoken words, though he could imitate nearly any
bird and could hear, smell, and feel almost anything that happened on top of the mountain.

The voices grew louder and clearer. The young man began
to think about his appearance. What did he look like? It had
been years since he had bathed properly or shaved. Would his
unkempt appearance frighten these people? He ran to the spring,
rinsed his body with cool water and smoothed back his hair
with his fingers. A few feet from the bubbling spring was a
small pool where a badger had built a dam of mud and branches.
He hurried to the pool, bent over, and stared at his reflection
in the still, calm water. How he had changed! His body was
hard and weathered from the many long winters on the mountain. He was lean like a deer, and his skin was as shiny and
clear as the stream. His hair was long and tangled, nearly to
his waist. His face was hidden somewhere behind a tangled
gray beard that held little twigs and bits of debris, as though
it were being readied for a bird's nest.

When he returned to his hut the strangers were already there,
seated outside on the large rocks. They said nothing; for several minutes the travelers and the old man just looked at each
other, sharing the silence of the mountain, the dance of the
wind, the music of rustling trees. The travelers offered him a
few special provisions from below and watched in amusement

as he tasted, smelled, and rubbed each object as though it were a precious stone.

Then they told the story of their own long, difficult journey up the mountain: how they had begun their ascent many years ago, frail and near death, hoping to find the famous old man who might be able to cure them of their terrible illnesses. And now, at last, after much hardship and suffering, they were here and overjoyed finally to meet this old man they had heard so much about, the one famous for curing people of incurable diseases. Though now, happily, they had no need for his services, for the long, difficult journey had restored them to perfect health.

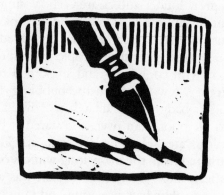

Appendixes

Appendix A

Rate Yourself Health Quiz

- Score each question according to the rating given. You may want to record your score on the Rate Yourself Scorecard on page 139.
- The total score will then indicate your rating, page 141.
- Note that questions 2, 3, 5, 10, and 15 have higher maximum scoring. These are the foundation stones of true health and are called Foundation Questions.
- The discussion within each question is important to help you select the most accurate rating. The whole family is encouraged to participate.
- If you prefer, just use the pinch and pat rating system.

1. Endurance

CAN YOU WALK VIGOROUSLY FOR ONE HOUR WITHOUT STOPPING? DO YOU DO THIS OR THE EQUIVALENT* REGULARLY?

This raises the question of physical endurance or stamina — how long your body can exert itself without getting overtired

* Exercise equivalents: Vigorous walking for 60 minutes — Vigorous bicycling (up and down hill) for 10 miles — Playful running for 30 minutes — Rapid swimming for

or strained. If, for instance, running to catch a bus or having to climb a flight of stairs leaves you huffing and puffing, you are most likely not in very good condition.

Just as important as the distance you can walk or the number of minutes you can skip rope or shovel is the regularity and the vigor with which you do it. How often do you walk each week, and is this walking done with real exertion, with oomph?

Rating

Can walk vigorously for an hour and do it, or the equivalent, regularly (three to four times per week)	give yourself 50 points, and a pat
Somewhere in between	20–40 points
Get tired just thinking about walking a mile	10 points, and a pinch

2. *Flexibility*

A: WHILE STANDING, FEET TOGETHER, HOW EASILY CAN YOU TOUCH YOUR HANDS TO THE FLOOR WITHOUT BENDING YOUR KNEES?
B: HOW EASY IS IT FOR YOU TO GIVE UP SOMETHING YOU'VE ALWAYS WANTED ONCE YOU GET IT?

The purpose of this question is to find out how easily and gracefully your body and mind respond when you're called

---

one-half mile — Jumping rope for 15 minutes — Vigorous manual labor (like chopping wood) for 30 minutes.

upon to be flexible. Flexible body plus flexible mind equals good health.

For example, when you want to lift furniture, do you run the risk of pulling a muscle or throwing your back out? When unexpected guests arrive or the stock market takes a sudden dip, can you deal with it?

Body flexibility and mind flexibility are two sides of the same coin. We all know how it feels to have a neck stiff from worry or a backache from a tense and frustrating situation.

Rating

A: Physical Flexibility

Palms easily rest on floor; as flexible as a child doing somersaults	give yourself 50 points, and a pat
Somewhere in between	20–40 points
Fingertips reach knees	10 points, and a pinch

B: Emotional Flexibility

Recover well from loss or change	50 points, and a pat
Somewhere in between	20–40 points
Easily upset; tend to be quite fragile	10 points, and a pinch

3. Relaxation

DO YOU TAKE TIME EACH DAY TO RELAX?

Are you one of those people who can never find time to relax? It is interesting that the word *relax* comes from the words *re,* meaning to do again, and *lax,* meaning loosen. Are you able to "make yourself loose again" each day, or do you get tighter and more tense as the day goes on?

At this point it's useful to describe the experience of a patient, Mrs. C.F., age sixty-two, who was brought to the author's clinic by her worried family. She had for many years complained of a tremor, insomnia, and anxiety. In fact, she was a persistent worrier and had become so accustomed to worrying that it had become a "natural" part of her life. She seldom allowed herself the freedom to relax. She liked going to the opera, but she worried that she would fall asleep during the performance, so she always gave her tickets away. It became clear that going to the opera was exactly the "medicine" she needed. When the next opera came around, she followed our prescription to go with a friend and allowed herself to fall asleep.

Later, at a follow-up visit, she reported that the opportunity to let go again had been well worth the part she'd missed in *Madame Butterfly*. Clinically, her body was less tense, her sleep had improved, and the tremor had subsided. And most important, she had relearned to re-lax.

Rating

Allow yourself to become as relaxed as a kitten napping in the sun, every day	give yourself 100 points, and a pat
Somewhere in between	20–90 points
Often as tense as a tightrope without getting a chance to relax	10 points, and a pinch

4. *Overeating*

DO YOU OVEREAT?

Overeating greatly diminishes our chances of enjoying good health. Giving our bodies more food than they need is like adding too rich a mixture of fuels to our automobile engines: after a while they are unable to utilize this fuel and operate less efficiently.

The amount of food our bodies need is a product of how much food we are able to burn up, how well we assimilate the food, our level of health, etc. A person who walks three miles a day, for example, will burn up more energy than a person whose life is less active. And what's more, the more active person will utilize the food better.

The amount of food our minds let us think we need depends on other factors. A person who is nervous and has a lot of problems may not feel adequately nourished no matter how much he or she eats, whereas a person who is calm and easily satisfied may be well nourished on a modest amount of food.

Rating

Eat modestly and always leave the table feeling slightly hungry	give yourself 50 points, and a pat
Somewhere in between	20–40 points
Constantly eating, yet seldom feel like you've had enough to eat	10 points, and a pinch

5. *Elimination*

IS ELIMINATION EASY AND REGULAR?

Although many will understand elimination to mean bowel elimination, it should be remembered that there are other important means of elimination: the kidneys and bladder, skin and sweat glands, lungs, and, very much overlooked, the emotions. In regard to emotional elimination, an interesting family case history might serve to illustrate the point.

A certain family was experiencing great pain upon the loss of a close relative. Their suffering was in silence and grew in intensity. When they were seen at the clinic, the ice broke when the children began to cry. This released a flood of tears from all and later much relief from the physical complaints that had initially brought them to see the doctor. This letting go of emotional tension was an important elimination of pent-up emotional toxins.

Good elimination is often overlooked. ✳ Under conditions of normal good health we should enjoy a bowel movement corresponding to every complete meal that we eat. In general, if we eat three full meals a day, we should have three bowel movements. Even though there are individual differences, those who become healthier and more relaxed will have easier and more frequent bowel movements; our bodies will extract the nutrients they need and elimination will be quick and easy.

Rating

A: Bowel Elimination

Your movements are as frequent and as regular as clockwork — without laxatives	give yourself 50 points, and a pat

Somewhere in between	20–40 points
Bowel movements are irregular, often very loose or very hard; must strain to move bowels	10 points, and a pinch

B: Emotional Elimination

Able to discharge emotional tension without hurting self or others	give yourself 50 points, and a pat
Somewhere in between	20–40 points
Have great difficulty discharging feelings in a constructive way	10 points, and a pinch

6. *Posture*

DO YOU SLOUCH?

Are you one of those people who always need something to lean on? When you enter a room, do you automatically seek out a convenient chair, cushion, sofa, or wall on which to prop yourself?

A body that fits together well can maintain good posture without being propped up. Such a body has the feeling and appearance of ease and lightness. It moves gracefully, does not tire easily, and rests comfortably, ready to spring into action when it is needed — like a cat.

Good posture is important to good health: it affects our breathing, vitality, and attitude. When our bodies are straight and tall, we breathe easier, have more energy, and feel more positive.

How can poor posture become good posture? Throughout

this book there are reminders to stand and sit straight: while bathing, eating, walking, reading this sentence — whatever we are doing. By becoming more aware of our posture and making an effort to improve it, we will be taking an important step toward better health.

Rating

You have good posture; don't need props to lean on; don't tend to slouch	give yourself 50 points, and a pat
Somewhere in between	20–40 points
Slouch much of the time	10 points, and a pinch

7. Body Weight

ARE YOU COMFORTABLE WITH THE DISTRIBUTION OF YOUR BODY WEIGHT?

Is there a scale in your bathroom? Do you stand on it very carefully, hoping it will not think you are too heavy or too light? And even if you are satisfied that your body weight is correct, is it distributed right?

There are many different beliefs about what is the right body weight for each of us. Often it is the ease with which we fit into our clothes. Haven't we all, at one time or another, heard someone say, "I'm going to lose weight until I can fit into a size twelve again"? For some it is a matter of fitting into a certain size; others may be satisfied with their weight because they consider themselves large-boned or small-boned.

Ultimately, of course, we know when we are carrying more weight than is necessary. We don't need a scale, mirror, or insurance chart to tell us we are getting plump here and there; we can feel it.

Rating

As sleek as a deer	give yourself 50 points, and a pat
Somewhere in between	20–40 points
Tend to have lumps and sags here and there	10 points, and a pinch

8. *Abdomen*

IS THERE SAGGING IN THE ABDOMEN?

Strong abdominal muscles are a cornerstone of good health, and a sagging abdomen is often a sign of weak abdominal muscles. Good posture and breathing, proper digestion and elimination, a relaxed and flexible spine, and well-toned internal organs are all benefits of a strong abdomen.

An evaluation of good abdominal muscles is the following test. Lie on your back, arms at sides. Keeping your legs straight, without bending your knees, lift your legs twelve inches in the air. Can you hold them there for thirty seconds?

Rating

Can grasp less than one-half inch below the belly button, using thumb and forefinger	give yourself 50 points, and a pat
Somewhere in between	20–40 points
If you're carrying around a spare tire	10 points, and a pinch

9. Chill

DO YOU CHILL EASILY?

If you chill easily, frequently catch colds when the weather changes, cannot tolerate cool water and cool air on your skin, and find that your hands and feet get cold quickly, your circulation is in need of a tonic.

Poor circulation means blood is not adequately reaching the different parts of your body. Without this continuous supply of fresh blood, your body is not getting the oxygen it needs to build new, healthy cells, to maintain a high level of resistance, to keep you vibrant and full of pep.

Rosy-cheeked children are constant proof of the glowing benefits of good circulation: a tolerance of sudden changes in weather, snug hands and feet, and a quick recovery from the occasional cold.

Rating

Can easily tolerate low temperatures
give yourself 50 points, and a pat

Somewhere in between
20–40 points

Can't tolerate low temperatures at all; can never get close enough to the heater
10 points, and a pinch

10. *Sleep and Stress*

DO YOU ENJOY A GOOD NIGHT'S SLEEP AND
WAKE UP FULLY RESTED — WITHOUT TAKING
SLEEPING PILLS?

The telltale signs of someone having increasing difficulty coping with stress are fingernail biting, picking at the skin or scalp, a drawn face, and, most important of all, poor sleep.

Rating

Wake up full of vim and vigor — every day	give yourself 100 points, and a pat
Somewhere in between	20–90 points
Have difficulty sleeping at night; often tired during the day	10 points, and a pinch

11. *Common Ailments*

HOW OFTEN DO YOU HAVE COMMON COMPLAINTS,
THE EVERYDAY AILMENTS MOST OF US REGARD AS
"NORMAL" (HEADACHES, STOMACH UPSET,
BACKACHE, SINUS CONGESTION, CONSTIPATION,
ETC.)?

Occasionally we all get a few minor ailments; however, when they occur repeatedly we should listen to these signals of failing health.

Rating

Seldom troubled by everyday complaints	give yourself 50 points, and a pat
Somewhere in between	20–40 points
Pharmacist's best customer	10 points, and a pinch

12. *Toxins*

ARE YOU EXPOSED REGULARLY TO KNOWN TOXINS SUCH AS CLEANING FLUIDS, DYES, RADIOACTIVE MATERIALS, SMOKE, X-RAYS, HIGH NOISE LEVELS, ETC.?

The list of known disease-related toxins could easily fill several books. Every week a new substance is banned, modified, or reexamined for its potentially harmful effects. As it becomes more and more difficult to avoid contact with these toxins, whether in the country or the city, it behooves us to minimize our exposure to them as well as raise our physical resistance. If we have low resistance, even mild exposure may seriously affect our health. On the other hand, if our resistance is strong, we stand a better chance of remaining healthy.

Rating

As exposure to toxins is difficult to measure and control, give yourself a pinch and a score of zero — a reminder that even the most careful among us are exposed each day to more and more forms of pollution.

13. *Excess and Moderation*

ARE YOU LIVING A LIFE OF EXCESS?

Who can say what excess is? What are the boundaries between moderation and excess for each individual? When does enough become too much? At what point does a person who exercises begin to suffer from overexercise?

These are difficult questions. For one person a couple of beers a day is moderate, for another it is excessive. For one person running a mile is child's play, for the next it is an ordeal. If smoking, for example, contributes to your nervous irritability, coughing, and sputum, it is excessive no matter how many cigarettes you actually smoke.

Rating

Yes, I know when I've had enough	give yourself 50 points, and a pat
Somewhere in between	20–40 points
More is never quite enough	10 points, and a pinch

14. *Satisfaction with Health*

ARE YOU SATISFIED WITH YOUR HEALTH AS IT IS NOW?

For some of us it doesn't take much to be satisfied: avoidance of major illness and only an occasional cold may be a high enough level of health. Others will not be content with anything less than vibrant health. And many are satisfied only because they do not yet realize that higher levels of health are available to them.

Whatever level of health we aspire to, be it the vitality of a child or just the avoidance of a debilitating disease, it must ultimately be satisfying to us.

Rating

Completely satisfied	give yourself 50 points, and a pat
Somewhere in between	20–40 points
Dissatisfied: with a strong motivation to improve, hence	50 points, and a pat!

15. Happiness

ARE YOU HAPPY?

Uncle Joe is happy when the sun shines. Aunt Mary prefers the rain. Brother John lives in Portugal, Brother Jim lives in Spain. Rain or shine, happiness is something each of us must define.

When things are not going well, when a smile is difficult to find, we are in need of encouragement. We need someone to take our hand and say, "You're a nice person. Keep doing whatever you do. Your life is meaningful. Don't worry. Be happy."

Happiness, like laughter, has often been called the best medicine. It has been known to cure illnesses that responded to no other treatment. Several years ago a French physician opened a happiness and laughter clinic where people came to learn how to laugh and enjoy themselves. The clinic was a great success.

RATE YOURSELF HEALTH QUIZ

Happiness is contagious. When we're happy we infect everyone around us with our good feelings.

Rating

Happy and content most of the time	give yourself 100 points, and a pat
Somewhere in between	20–90 points
A sad clown	10 points, and a pinch

Rate Yourself Scorecard

* Foundation Questions

	PINCHES	PATS	POINTS
1. Endurance			
*2. A: Flexibility (physical)			
*2. B: Flexibility (emotional)			
*3. Relaxation			
4. Overeating			
*5. A: Elimination (physical: bowel)			
*5. B: Elimination (emotional)			
6. Posture			
7. Body weight			
8. Abdomen			
9. Chill			
*10. Sleep and stress			
11. Common ailments			
12. Toxins			
13. Excess and moderation			
14. Satisfaction with health			
*15. Happiness			
TOTALS			

Rate Yourself Again in Six Months.
Rate Yourself Scorecard

*Foundation Questions	PINCHES	PATS	POINTS
1. Endurance			
*2. A: Flexibility (physical)			
*2. B: Flexibility (emotional)			
*3. Relaxation			
4. Overeating			
*5. A: Elimination (physical: bowel)			
*5. B: Elimination (emotional)			
6. Posture			
7. Body weight			
8. Abdomen			
9. Chill			
*10. Sleep and stress			
11. Common ailments			
12. Toxins			
13. Excess and moderation			
14. Satisfaction with health			
*15. Happiness			
TOTALS			

Your Health Rating

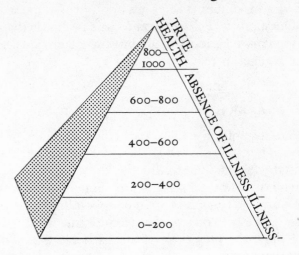

800–1000: EXCELLENT

You're near the top of the Pyramid of Health. I hope your high score has come from at least three good marks on the Foundation Questions (2, 3, 5, 10, and 15). These are the foundation stones of true health.

As you already know, good health requires everyday practice — there is no limit to flexibility, vitality, and happiness. Even though you may have scored well, chances are there are still areas where you need improvement. You might, for example, be very flexible and happy but have a weak abdomen. This book will teach you how to improve your health, and perhaps more important, how to maintain it.

600–800: HIGH AVERAGE

You've obviously scored maximum on some questions, but not enough all the way through. Look at questions 2, 3, 5, 10, and

15 again — these are important health areas where improvement is usually needed.

Scoring a maximum (100 points) on just two more Foundation Questions will elevate you to true health. Perhaps just improving your relaxation or elimination will do it. This book will help you get there.

400–600: AVERAGE

This means it's unlikely you've scored high on the Foundation Questions (2, 3, 5, 10, and 15), the most important building blocks in the Pyramid of Health.

Likewise, if your total score on the Foundation Questions was 300 or more, you have scored disappointingly low on the other ten questions. You're within reach of true health — reach for it! Follow the prescriptions in this book, and you'll be pleasantly surprised as your health score improves.

200–400: BELOW AVERAGE

You're at the bottom of the Absence of Illness category. At best, you've scored well on only one of the Foundation Questions (2, 3, 5, 10, and 15), the most important building blocks in the Pyramid of Health. Likewise, your performance on the rest of the evaluation is no more than average.

Your health pyramid is on a foundation that needs strengthening. Follow the prescriptions in this book.

LESS THAN 200: POOR

Your Foundation score is critically low. These are the building blocks to good health.

Your performance on the rest of the evaluation was also

poor. Even though you may not have the classic symptoms of illness, your health pyramid is weak and in danger of collapse.

Read this book very carefully. You *have* the tools for improving your health, and this book can teach you how to use them.

Congratulations! You have completed the Health Quiz and should now have a better understanding of your true health at this time.

If you're glowing from all the pats, keep up the good work! You have undoubtedly retained many of the healthy attributes of childhood.

If you're sore from so many pinches, please do not be discouraged. This book will give you the tools you need to recover and restore the disciplines of good health.

And if you're like most people who take this quiz, your health and vitality is probably somewhere between a pinch and a pat: you consider yourself healthy simply because you're not sick.

Is this enough? Are you really satisfied with living free from illness and disease, but without true vitality and vigor? If you're not completely satisfied and would like more — without the expense and time of pills, health gadgets, special diets, and medications — then read this book carefully. Each chapter is a prescription for good health. When you take these prescriptions regularly and enthusiastically, you'll soon rediscover some old childhood friends: clear skin, good digestion, and a good night's sleep — sure signs that you're on the road to true health.

Appendix B

Health Improvement Programs

Exercise Notes

· While doing the exercises that follow, always keep your knees
  slightly flexed, never locked.

- If your back hurts or is weak, save the exercises that twist until you are fitter.
- If you have a medical problem that limits your ability to move, consult your doctor before beginning the program.

1. *General Flexibility*

These movements are to be done slowly and rhythmically. At no time should you force your body into a position. Avoid fast, brusque movements, and always keep your knees slightly bent.

As these movements become easier, add more repetitions and hold each position longer. When you get to the last exercise, try them in reverse order, beginning with number 10 and ending with number 1.

These movements serve as a general tonic. If you do them carefully and regularly, they will tone and strengthen your muscles and contribute greatly to your good health.

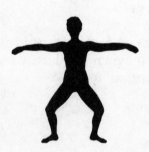

STRETCH 1

- Stand with your arms held out at shoulder level.
- Turn your toes out, keeping your feet flat on the floor.

- Keeping your spine straight, bend your knees as far as possible without lifting heels.
- Try to keep your knees directly over your toes.
- If balancing is difficult, hold on to any sturdy piece of furniture.
- Repeat several times.

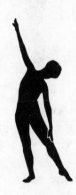

STRETCH 2

- Stand with your feet about 12 inches apart.
- Swing your right hip out to the right side as far as possible.
- Slide your left hand down your left leg as far as possible.
- Keep your spine straight.
- Reverse to the other side.

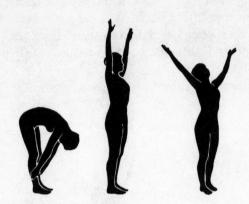

STRETCH 3

- Stand with your legs shoulder width apart, knees slightly flexed.
- While exhaling through the nose, slowly bend forward from the waist and clasp your knees or ankles, whichever is easier. Do not strain.
- While inhaling through the nose, come up slowly, raising your arms over your head.
- Open your arms wide and lean back slightly, again taking care not to strain.

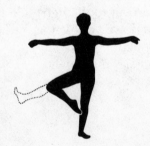

STRETCH 4

- Extend your arms at shoulder level, holding lightly to a support such as a sturdy piece of furniture or a wall.

- Keeping your back straight and your pelvis facing forward, slide your foot along the inside of your standing leg, bringing it to a comfortable height.
- At the top of the movement, straighten your leg in the air, flexing your toes and tightening the entire leg.
- Hold, then bring your leg down with the knee straight.
- Repeat with each leg several times.

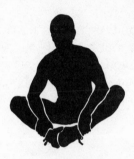

STRETCH 5

- Sit on the floor with your knees out to the side and your heels together.
- Place your hands on your ankles and gently pull your upper body forward toward your feet, bending from the waist. Keep your back straight, and do not strain.
- Hold this position for ten seconds, breathing slowly in and out through the nose.
- Repeat several times.

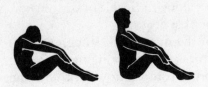

STRETCH 6

- Sit with your knees bent.
- Clasp your knees and round your back. Pull your stomach in forcibly, dropping your head.
- Pull the middle of your body back, away from the knees.
- Flatten your back and lift your head high.
- Repeat several times.

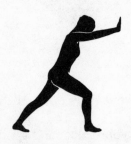

STRETCH 7

- Hold on to any heavy piece of furniture at about shoulder level.
- Bend your right leg as much as is comfortable.
- Step back with your left leg as far as comfortable, keeping that knee straight and your back flat. Try to keep both feet facing straight ahead, one in front of the other, and the back heel flat on the ground.
- Repeat with the other leg.

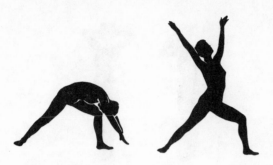

STRETCH 8

- Step forward on your left leg, bending your left knee as much as possible.
- Keep your back leg straight and lean as far forward and down as you can.
- Keeping the left leg in the bent position, bring your torso up, with your arms over your head, and bend back slightly.
- Repeat with the other leg.

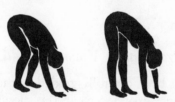

STRETCH 9

- Bend your knees and place your palms on the floor.
- Now try to straighten your knees without letting your hands come up off floor.
- Try to keep the spine straight, not rounded, and do not extend your legs all the way to the locked-knee position.
- Repeat several times.

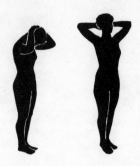

STRETCH 10

- Stand with your legs about shoulder width apart, knees slightly flexed, hands clasped behind your head.
- Exhaling through the nose, move your head slowly forward and down.
- Inhaling through the nose, slowly bring your head up, gently pulling your elbows apart as you come up.
- Repeat several times, moving slowly without jerking your head or neck.

2. *Program in Vigorous Walking*

This program has been carefully graded so that a person with no previous exercise experience can very slowly and gradually get into good physical condition. You should repeat each phase as long as necessary until you are strong enough to go on to the next phase. Be sure to walk in good posture.

Normal Walking and Vigorous Walking

FIRST PHASE

Days 1 and 3	Day 5	Day 7
Normal 5 minutes	Normal 15 minutes	Normal 15 minutes
Vigorous 1 minute	Vigorous 5 minutes	Vigorous 5 minutes
(Repeat for 30 minutes.)	Normal 10 minutes	Normal 15 minutes

SECOND PHASE

Normal 4 minutes	Normal 20 minutes	Normal 15 minutes
Vigorous 1 minute	Vigorous 10 minutes	Vigorous 15 minutes
(Repeat for 50 minutes.)	Normal 10 minutes	Normal 15 minutes

THIRD PHASE

Normal 3 minutes	Normal 20 minutes	Normal 15 minutes
Vigorous 1 minute	Vigorous 15 minutes	Vigorous 20 minutes
(Repeat for 50 minutes.)	Normal 15 minutes	Normal 15 minutes

FOURTH PHASE

Normal 3 minutes	Normal 20 minutes	Normal 15 minutes
Vigorous 1 minute	Vigorous 20 minutes	Vigorous 30 minutes
(Repeat for 30 minutes.)	Normal 20 minutes	Normal 15 minutes

FIFTH PHASE

Normal 2 minutes	Normal 15 minutes	Vigorous 60 minutes
Vigorous 1 minute	Vigorous 30 minutes	Normal to recover
(Repeat for 60 minutes.)	Normal 15 minutes	

3. *Improving Elimination and Firming Abdominal Muscles*

A. THE CAMEL

• Get on all fours. Let your abdomen relax toward the floor so that your lower spine bows slightly toward the floor also. As you do this, inhale so that you inflate the abdomen and chest.
• Now exhale fully, removing all the air from your lungs.
• Do not breathe in immediately. Instead, push your hands into the floor and arch your back. As you do so, suck your stomach in toward your spine. Pull your stomach and abdomen in firmly. Hold for five to ten seconds without straining.
• Relax the abdomen back toward the floor and inhale deeply.
• Repeat three to five times. With some practice you will be able to hold the posture, with the abdomen drawn in, for fifteen to thirty seconds.

B. ROCKING HORSE

• Lie on your back on a soft, well-cushioned mat. Grasp your ankles, raise your knees to your chest, and rock gently back and forth — head to toe — a few times. Breathe through your nose while rocking.
• Stop rocking and hold your knees as close as possible to your chest.
• Slowly bring your bent knees toward your forehead. Do not strain; just bring them as near as you can.
• Hold this position, knees to forehead, for several seconds, breathing normally. Then, exhaling through your nose, lower the knees and relax.
• Repeat three times.

4. *The Magic Five*

MAGIC ONE: YAWN AND STRETCH

• Stand tall. Clench your fists and press them against your chest. Very slowly raise your arms into the air, opening your mouth and fists at the same time. Open your mouth as wide as you can and try to yawn. Stretch your fingers out as far as possible.

• Now slowly bring your arms back to your chest, pulling your fingers in until your fists are clenched again.

• Repeat eight to ten times, yawning and stretching in this manner. Think of yourself as a flower, petals opening to the morning sun.

MAGIC TWO: BUTTERFLY

• Stand in good posture, knees slightly flexed.

• Clasp your hands in back of your neck, fingers laced together. Inhale slowly through the nose, at the same time pulling your elbows back as far as is comfortable, like the wings of a butterfly.

• Now bend slowly forward, exhaling through your nose, bending your elbows, and touching your chest with your chin.

• Begin inhaling again, pulling your elbows open and back until your butterfly wings are fully spread.

• Repeat twelve times, breathing slowly and rhythmically through your nose, expanding and contracting your chest with each inhalation and exhalation.

• Move gently at all times, without jerking your head or neck.

MAGIC THREE: BIRD

• Stand with your arms stretched out on either side of your body like the wings of a bird.

- Keeping your back straight and your knees slightly bent, begin slowly tilting your wings to the left, dropping your left hand toward your left side and raising your right hand up over your head until it is perfectly vertical. Allow your head to move gently with your arms and follow the arc of your wings. Pause in this position for several seconds.
- Now slowly begin tilting your wings to the right, continuing until your left hand is directly over your head and your right hand is at your right side. Allow your head to move gently with your arms and follow the arc of your wings. Pause in this position for several seconds, then begin tilting again toward the left.
- Do this six times, going slowly from side to side, taking care not to jerk your head or neck.

MAGIC FOUR: SHOULDER SHRUG

- Sit or stand with your arms hanging relaxed at your sides. Raise both shoulders at the same time as though you were trying to touch your shoulders to your ears.
- Now move your shoulders forward, then down, then toward your back, then back to where you started. The movements should be that of a smooth circle.
- Reverse the direction of the movement and do the same thing.
- Repeat five to ten times in each direction.

MAGIC FIVE: SOCK LIFT

- Take the socks you are going to wear and drop them on the floor. Reach down with your right foot and curl your toes around one of the socks. Lift it into the air about twelve inches, squeezing hard. Open your toes, relax your grip, and allow the sock to drop. Do this six times.
- Now do the same thing with your left foot six times. With

some practice you will be able to sit on a chair or on the edge of a bed and pick up both socks simultaneously using both feet.

5. Exercise Breaks for the Office

The movements below are especially beneficial for those who spend long periods of time sitting. They take very little space or time, and if done regularly will make your work more pleasant and efficient.

If possible, loosen your belt, tie, etc., remove your shoes, and find a small area in front of an open window.

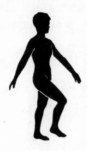

JOGGING IN PLACE

Begin by alternately lifting your left heel, then your right heel. Gradually change to light jogging. Try to keep your arms relaxed and moving naturally while jogging.

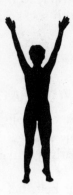

STRETCHING AND YAWNING

Stretch your arms upward, going up on tiptoes as you do so. Reach toward the ceiling and yawn, then let your arms fall, and shake your shoulders.

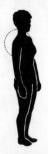

SHOULDER ROLLING

Raise your shoulders one at a time, then pull them backward, then relax. Continue alternately rolling and relaxing your shoulders. After rolling several times, shake them one at a time, then relax.

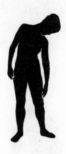

SIDE BENDING

Stand with your feet comfortably apart, about shoulder width. Slowly bend to the left and hold the position. Then bend slowly to the right and hold. Let your weight pull you toward the floor on each side.

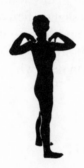

SIDE TURNING

Stand with your feet shoulder width apart. Bend your elbows so that your fingertips touch your shoulders. Keeping your feet pointed straight ahead, slowly and gently turn the upper part of your body to the left. Hold this position, without straining, three to five seconds. Now slowly pivot and move in the opposite direction, assuming the same position on the right side. Hold, without straining, three to five seconds. Continue moving slowly and rhythmically from side to side, allowing your head and eyes to move with the upper body. Do not jerk or strain.

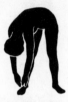

FRONT BENDING

Stand with your feet shoulder width apart. Clasp your hands in front of your body and gently lean forward, bending from the waist. Keep the knees slightly flexed. First lean toward your left leg, then straighten and lean toward your right leg. Do not jerk or pull the body forward. Let gravity do the work. Try to relax your arms and neck while bending.

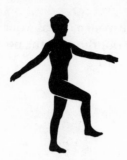

JUMPING/HOPPING

Hop alternately, twice on one foot, then twice on the other. Keep your knees high. Finish with a moderate jog in place.

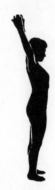

STRETCHING AND RELAXING

Stand with your feet shoulder width apart, hands at sides. Swing your arms slowly forward and upward until they are as far in back of your head as is comfortable. Hold several seconds in that position, without straining.

Now let your arms fall slowly forward, bending your knees slightly as they fall. Pull your arms up and as far in back of your body as comfortable. Hold several seconds, without straining.

Breathe in through your nose as your arms move forward and upward. Breathe out through the nose as your arms move downward and backward.

Appendix C

Short Essays on Nutrition

1. Fiber

In recent years fiber has been much publicized as one of the great nutritional "discoveries" of the century. What exactly is fiber? What does it do? How do we make sure we are getting enough?

WHAT IS FIBER?

Fiber comes exclusively from plants — cereals, vegetables, fruits, nuts, and seeds. The amount of fiber varies greatly from plant to plant and also within a given plant depending on the time of year. While being an edible material, fiber is technically considered nonnutritive because it is not readily assimilable by the intestinal tract.

WHAT DOES FIBER DO?

Fiber tends to improve and facilitate bowel movement. Though fiber varies greatly, *in general, increasing the amount of fiber increases the amount and bulk of stool, accelerates stool transit time, and increases the motor activity of the colon, thereby promoting and facilitating elimination. Recent studies indicate that increased intake of dietary fiber offers some degree of protection from many chronic disorders, especially those related to the colon.*

HOW MUCH FIBER IS NEEDED?

Although estimates vary on how much fiber is needed for good health, most researchers agree that Western diets are generally low in fiber. *Most people eating a normal Western diet can double their daily fiber intake with beneficial results. This can be done by eating more high-fiber and bran cereals, whole grains (rice, millet, buckwheat, rye, etc.), beans, raw fruits and

*These studies also point out that while Western diet is low in fiber, it is also high in sucrose, refined carbohydrates, animal fats, and protein, factors that may contribute to numerous diseases. For further information on fiber, see "Fiber," A. Mendeloff et al., in *Nutrition in Disease,* Ross Laboratories, 1978.

vegetables, and nuts. For best results, increase the amount of fiber slowly, giving your body a chance to get accustomed to the bulkier food. Most people report feeling better because of improved elimination. Try it and find out for yourself.

2. Complete Protein Through a Simple Food Combination

Protein provides the necessary material for building and replacing tissues and cells. The amount of protein an individual requires is determined by a host of factors, including age, amount of physical activity, body size and build, and level of stress encountered in daily life.

Protein-rich foods include beans, cheese, eggs, whole grains, pulses (lentils, peas, etc.), nuts, seeds, and leafy dark green vegetables such as spinach and kale.

Complete proteins — those containing the eight essential amino acids — are produced by a simple food combination: add one-quarter cup of beans, lentils, or peas to each cup of whole grain, such as rice, millet, or corn. This simple, natural combination is found in native diets throughout the world: soybeans and rice in Asia; dal and chapatis in India; black beans and corn in South America; tempeh and rice in Indonesia; corn, squash, and beans among Native Americans.

3. The Sugar Story

Sugar is a primary body fuel and is found in all foods, to varying degrees. If allowed to do so, the body will manufacture the sugar it needs from the food that is put in: it extracts natural sugar from fresh vegetables and fruits and transforms complete carbohydrates (whole grains) into sugar. The body is like a sugar factory, continually making and processing sugar for its own use.

Whole grains or complex carbohydrates contain large quantities of sugar in a form the body needs and can utilize. Examples of complex carbohydrates include corn, brown rice, barley, millet, oats, and wheat. These are loaded with natural sugar, which is why many sweeteners and candies are made directly from whole grain.

Sugar is also present in all fresh raw fruits and vegetables: celery, carrots, corn, beets, lettuce, peas, etc. This accounts for their sweetness, especially if eaten shortly after harvest. The body extracts sugar from these foods in much the same way it extracts sugar from complex carbohydrates.

SUGAR CRAVINGS

When the body does not get enough complex carbohydrates and fresh raw fruits and vegetables from which to extract its own sugar, it starts looking for other sugar sources to run the factory and produce energy. Under this sugar-deficient condition it finds more refined sugars, the kind found in processed breakfast cereals, soda pop, alcohol, bread, pastry, etc.

Sugar in this form satisfies the body's need for sugar, but only for a short time; refined sugars, because they do not require conversion and work by the body, burn very quickly and must constantly be replaced. This rapid burning, the result of refined sugar being dumped into the bloodstream, leads to sugar "highs" but also sugar addiction. This craving for sugar, and the accompanying symptoms when we don't get it (depression, irritability, sluggishness) is commonly known as hypoglycemia or low blood sugar. Relief and satisfaction are generally short-lived and come only from eating more and more sugar.

Natural sugars — those found in dried fruits, fruit juices, honey, molasses, and maple syrup — meet the body's needs for sugar but, like refined sugars, are quickly burned and lead to further sugar cravings. ✳While these natural sugars are preferable to refined sugars, they are very concentrated and lead to hypoglycemic reactions similar to those brought on by refined sugars. Many people eating "natural" diets and using large quantities of concentrated natural sugars are actually hooked on sweeteners, even though they are more natural ones.

HOW TO KICK THE SUGAR HABIT

- Eat a generous supply of whole grains every day (see Bread and Cooked Whole Grains, page 168) supplemented with fresh raw fruits and vegetables, so your body will once more learn to draw the sugar it needs out of natural food.
- Eat honey and other natural sweeteners in moderation, diluted with water. Honey is highly concentrated; a honeybee makes only one-half teaspoon of honey in its entire lifetime of work!
- Dilute all fruit and vegetable juices fifty-fifty with fresh water.
- Begin juicing fruits and vegetables with your own champion juicer — your teeth. Thorough mastication slowly draws the sugar out of the food, dilutes it so it's not too sweet, and prepares it for a happy journey through the body.
- Reconstitute all dried fruit by soaking for at least twenty-four hours in fresh water.
- Introduce children to whole grains at an early age so their little bodies will learn the art of manufacturing natural sugars. The first food after mother's milk should be made from whole grain, preferably oat milk, followed by oat cream made from ground oats. ✳Oat milk, which has natural sweetness and nutrients very similar to mother's milk, is made by soaking freshly ground oats (macerate whole oat groats in a

blender) in water. Use one-quarter cup oats for each quart of fresh water. Soak overnight.

4. Bread and Cooked Whole Grains

Many people include a liberal amount of whole-grain bread in their diet, thinking they are getting the nutrition they need from whole grains. Unfortunately, this is no longer true.

Not too many years ago bread was baked only a few minutes after it was milled into flour. Under present-day conditions most grain is milled into flour, then stored, shipped, and made into bread at a later time.

This is an important difference. *Extensive research on nutrition has shown that once a grain is milled, it begins to deteriorate nutritionally within a few minutes.

What does this mean for modern-day health? Simply this: the whole-grain bread we buy or make ourselves from purchased flour, although superior to white or enriched bread, does not contain the vitamins and minerals needed to build healthy bodies and teeth.

This does not mean we should stop eating whole-grain bread. It means that in order to get the full nutritional bounty from grains and cereals, we should endeavor to eat them before they are milled, or make a special effort to buy or make whole-grain bread that is cooked shortly after milling.

Eating whole grains before they are milled — that is, cooked grains such as rice, millet, buckwheat, corn, and oats — will ensure that our bodies get the nourishment they need from whole grains. Eating cooked whole grains has other advantages. Because cooked whole grain is coarser than most bread, it requires more chewing, which strengthens our teeth and gums. Furthermore, eating whole grains puts more bulk and fiber in our diets, thereby improving and facilitating elimination.

Those who want to eat the staff of life when it is most nutritious should consider obtaining a grain mill so they can grind the flour just prior to baking. Alternatively, soft grains such as buckwheat, millet, and oats can be milled in most electric blenders, then made into fresh bread.

Afterword

I PAUSE NOW, putting my shovel aside in favor of the pen. This very day I have been laboring in the open air, turning the soil, coaxing it here and there as I prepare the foundation of a new dwelling, the seedbed of a new garden. How similar these two tools, the shovel and the pen: one capable of turning the earth, preparing it for growth and change, the other capable of turning the mind, preparing it for growth and change.

Words and ideas, like seeds, require very special conditions if they are to germinate. Some, it seems, spring up almost immediately and grow quickly and vigorously, while others lie dormant for months or even years before coming to life. When they finally do appear, it is often when we least expect them. We may be driving down a crowded freeway or lying in a tub of hot water when an idea planted long before will suddenly burst forth — like a flower opening inside our head.

The human organism is a remarkable instrument. With the foot, for example, we can kick a ball across a grassy field. With the hand we can throw a stone across a stream or a river. With the nose we can smell the aroma of a delicate flower. With the ear we can hear the sound of an insect beating its wings. With the eye we can see stars on the distant horizon. With the mind we can cross oceans and continents, traverse generations and ideas, journey where there are no borders except those we choose to create. The boundaries of the human spirit are truly limitless.

True health, like a gentle breeze or a honeybee, dusts and pollinates everything and everyone it touches. Healthy water, for example, demands that we safeguard the streams and rivers from which that water flows. Healthy, vibrant food requires healthy, uncontaminated soil. Proper oxygenation of the lungs demands not only long walks but also clean, unpolluted air. A peaceful social environment in which to raise healthy children requires good communication with other peoples of the world, a cultivation and appreciation of similarities and common interests.

In short, the true goal of health, and this simple book, is to improve the tilth of the human condition, to encourage you, dear reader, to make the earth a little better for having trod upon it.

A Few Inspiring Books

Sally and Lucian Berg, *The Vegetarian Gourmet,* Herder and Herder, 1971.

M. Bircher-Benner, *The Prevention of Incurable Disease,* James Clark and Company, 1969.

George Bizet, "Children's Games," Nonesuch Records.

Paul Bragg, *South Sea Culture of the Abdomen,* Health Science Press, 1975.

Berit Brattnas, *Better Bodies — Better Health,* Swedish Information Service.

Thornton W. Burgess, *Old Mother West Wind,* Little, Brown and Company, 1910.

Edward Carpenter, *Civilization: Its Cause and Cure,* Tao Books.

Rachel Carr, *Be a Frog, or a Bird, or a Tree,* Doubleday, 1973.

C. Ward Crampton, *Physical Exercise for Daily Use,* P. F. Collier, 1929.

Gertrude Enelow, *Body Dynamics,* Information Incorporated, 1960.

Mahatma Gandhi, *The Natural Cure,* Navajivan Publishing House, 1954.

David Grayson, *Adventures in Contentment,* Phillips Publishing Company, 1906.

Grace Halsell, *Los Viejos, Secrets of Long Life From the Sacred Valley,* Rodale Press, 1976.

Edmund Jacobson, *You Must Relax,* McGraw-Hill, 1934.

Gertrude Alice Kay, *Helping the Weatherman,* P. F. Volland Company, 1920.

Leslie and McClure, *Exercises for the Elderly,* University of Iowa, 1975.

Juliette Levy, *Nature's Children,* Schocken, 1971.

Hugh Lofting, *Doctor Doolittle, A Treasury,* J. P. Lippincott, 1967.

Rabbi David Miller, *The Secret of Happiness,* Committee of Rabbi David Miller Foundation, 1937.

Helen and Scott Nearing, *Living the Good Life,* Schocken Books, 1970.

A FEW INSPIRING BOOKS

John Nash Ott, *Health and Light,* Devin-Adair Company, 1973.

Pierre Parodi, *The Use of Poor Means in Helping the Third World,* Greenleaf Books, 1964.

Weston Price, *Nutrition and Physical Degeneration,* Price-Pottenger Foundation, 1945.

C. W. Saleeby, *Sunlight and Health,* G. P. Putnam, 1924.

Florence Scovel Shinn, *The Secret Door to Success,* Gerald Rickard, 1941.

Johanna Spiri, *Heidi,* Grosset and Dunlap, 1927.

Rudolph Steiner, *Problems of Nutrition,* Anthroposophic Press, 1909.

Frank Stockman, *The Bee Man of Orn,* Holt, Rinehart, Winston, 1964.

Aaron Sussman and Ruth Goode, *The Magic of Walking,* Simon and Schuster, 1967.

E. B. Szekely, *Healing Waters,* Academy Books.

Ernst Van Aaken, *Van Aaken Method,* Runner's World, 1967.

Prescription
℞

For Health and Happiness at Any Age,
Take Daily as Directed

℞ 1

Upon rising, do a few gentle stretching exercises, breathing deeply through your nose.

℞ 2

Do some simple, practical thing with your hands. Work in the garden. Hang clothes on the line. Bake. Sew. Carve. Draw a picture for a friend.

℞ 3

Take a long, vigorous walk in the fresh air. Get to know flowers and trees, insects and animals, children and neighbors. Walk tall, in good posture.

℞ 4

Close your eyes. Relax. Take a nap. Give yourself a few minutes of complete relaxation every day.

℞ 5

Establish a harmonious rhythm of living. Go to bed before you are overtired. Rise before the sun is too high in the sky. Avoid taking on more work or responsibility than you can comfortably handle.

℞ 6

Actively work to preserve the beauty of the natural environment. Make the earth healthier for having trod upon it.

℞ 7

Think and act positively. Laughter, smiles, and kind words are powerful medicine. Feeling good is contagious. Infect other people with your health and happiness.

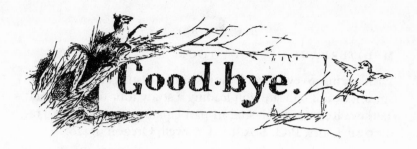

Good·bye.

Svevo Brooks, a European-trained educator and nutritionist, has been practicing common sense health care in both clinic and field for over twenty years. He has lived with and studied the traditional health practices of inhabitants of Africa, Asia, Latin America, the Caribbean, and the Mediterranean. A former professional athlete and elementary school teacher, he is a popular speaker on health, fitness, and environmental issues. His many interests include volunteer public service, gardening, beekeeping, and writing children's stories. *The Art of Good Living* was completed while the author was living on the Greek island of Kos, home of Hippocrates, the father of modern medicine.

LECTURES, SEMINARS, RADIO PROGRAM

If you would like to be notified when Svevo Brooks is speaking in your area, or if you are interested in helping to arrange a talk, workshop, or local radio broadcast of his "Common Sense Health Tips" program, please write to The Optimal Health Institute, 81900 Mahr Lane, Creswell, Oregon 97426.

MEDITERRANEAN STUDY TOUR

Each spring Svevo Brooks joins other distinguished and inspiring health educators in leading a study tour to Greece and Turkey. Readers interested in participating may contact Traditional Tours, P.O. Box 564, Creswell, Oregon 97426.

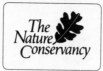
The
Nature
Conservancy

The Nature Conservancy is a 500,000-member international conservation organization committed to preserving natural diversity by finding and protecting lands and waters supporting the best examples of all elements of the natural world.

Since 1951, the Conservancy has protected more than 3.8 million acres in fifty states and helped protect millions more in Canada, Latin America, and the Caribbean.

Forests, wetlands, prairies, mountains, deserts, and islands — refuges for rare plants and threatened wildlife, places of special beauty — remain protected because the Conservancy and its members cared and acted quickly.

Our health is tied to the health of the environment in ways we are still exploring. Saving natural lands and waters must be a national priority if we are to leave the world a healthier place for future generations.

In this spirit, we (the author and the publisher) are supporting the work of The Nature Conservancy by contributing royalties from the sale of this book. We hope you will join us in this worthy effort.

- -

SB30000

Yes, I want to help The Nature Conservancy protect the natural world. Please enroll me as a member.

_____ I enclose $15 for one year's dues.
_____ I want to do more. Enclosed is an additional contribution of
　　　$_____.

Name_____

Address_____

City_____ State_____ ZIP_____

All contributions are tax deductible. The Nature Conservancy is a nonprofit, tax-exempt corporation under section 501(c)(3) of the Internal Revenue Code and is a publicly supported organization as defined in sections 170 (b)(1)(vi) and 509(a). Please make checks payable to The Nature Conservancy and mail to: Department SB30000, 1815 North Lynn Street, Arlington, VA 22209.